Dedication

This book is dedicated to all those who I have helped personally and helped me on my recovery journey and to the memory of those who are no longer with us.

Special Thanks

To my long suffering partner Samantha whose support has made this book possible? For putting up with my frustrations, self doubt and nonsense!

A special thank you has to go to **Laura Kirkham** one of our dedicated and enthusiastic volunteers who looks after our web site based directory maintaining it and updating it and with out who's help this book could not have been written.

Contents

Organisations

Introduction

This guide is for both those with existing mental health issues or those who are new to mental health and can be used both by the person with the issue or someone who is helping them on their journey to recovery.

Within these pages you will find help and information on what the causes and symptoms of poor mental health and illness can be.

Where you can get crisis support, national contact numbers for those not living in Manchester who can help you access local support and contact details for a 100 support agencies based here in Manchester some of which are run by the NHS, some by charities, some by voluntary organisations and some like Recovery Manchester that are non for profit social enterprises.

For each organisation you will find there contact information, what kind of support they give, if they are age or gender specific and when they are open.

We hope you will find the information helpful and useful and that it may help reduce your worry and your fears and put your mind at rest that you are not on your own, you don't have to suffer in silence and that help is there if you want it.

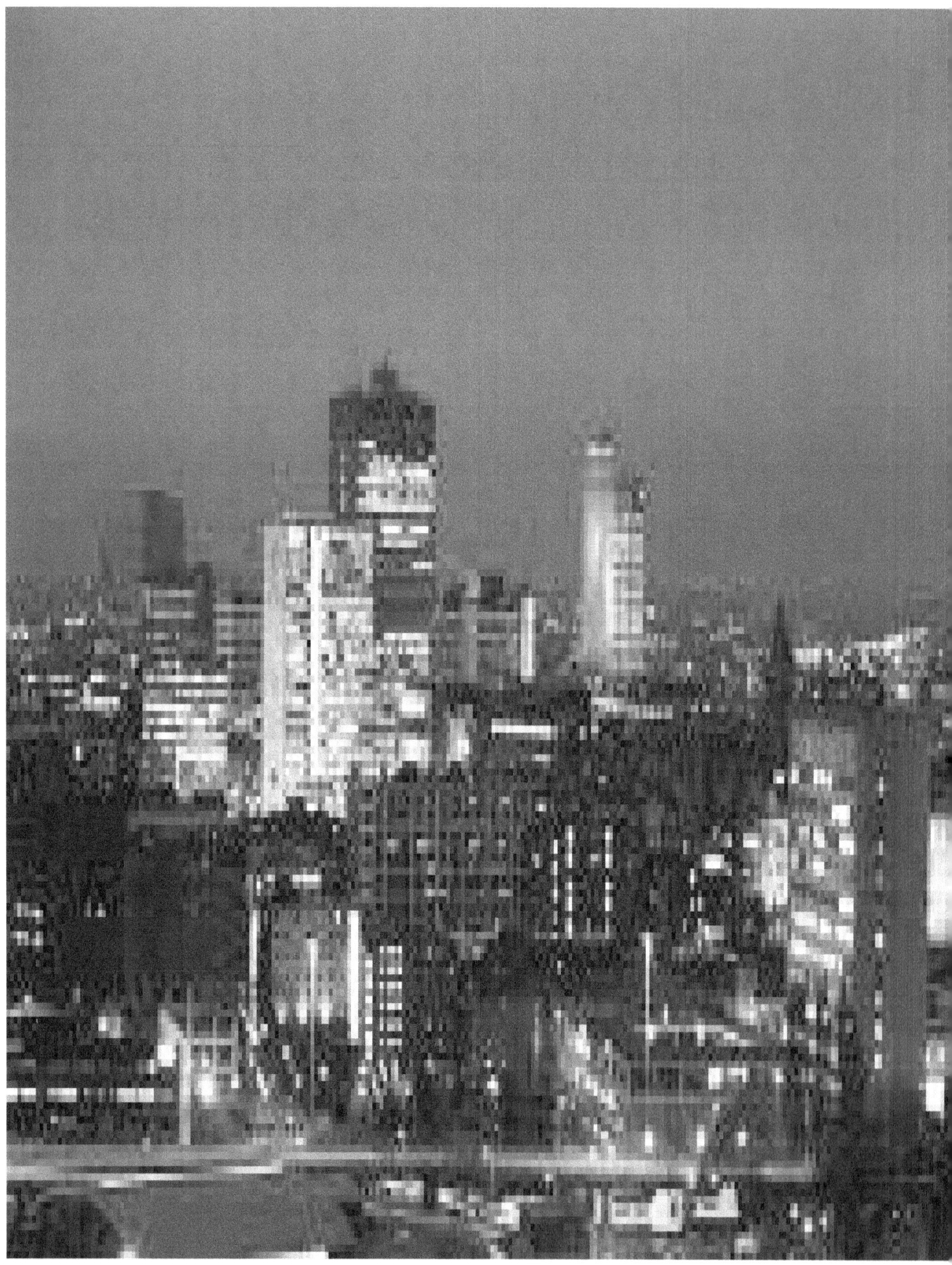

About Mental Health

What is mental health or illness? Some would say they are separate entities and some would say they are one in the same but there is a definition of what it is:

- Mental Health is anything that affects our way of thinking about our selves and others and the world we live in. (NIACE)

- Positive mental health means we can interact in the world in a "normal way"

- Poor mental health affects the way we function in society and day to day living and would make us therefore "abnormal"

In the UK there are nationally 1 in 5 people who will experience some kind of mental health issue in their life time and in some areas such as Manchester it can be as high as 1 in 3 which makes this type of illness as prevalent as Cancer or diabetes.

It is the biggest killer of young men and is rated in the top 5 of most serious illnesses by the World Health Organisation (WHO).

Globally there are more than 450 million people living with a mental health issue that's more than the entire population of the UK and the USA added together. Therefore being "abnormal" is more "normal" than you think??!!

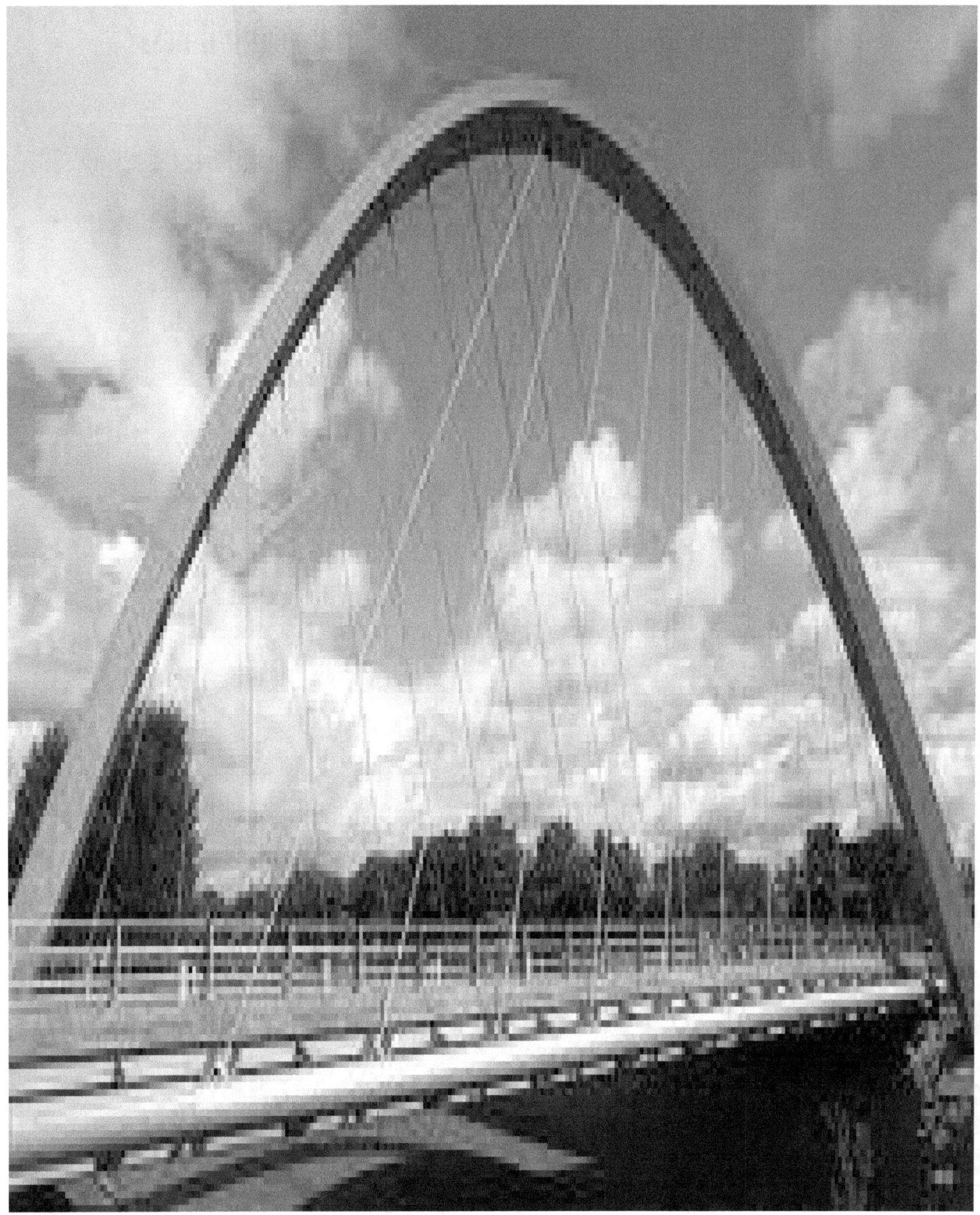

What are the causes of poor mental health/illness?

There are many causes of poor mental health/illness and for each person they will be different. Below is a list of some of the more common causes and it is far from an exhaustive list:

- It can be caused by a physical problem or illness.

- Lack of certain vitamins, minerals and hormones.

- Chemical imbalances within the brain e.g. too much of one or not enough and vice versa.

- Life events/trauma can also cause poor mental health this is sometimes referred to as a "product of their environment"

- Substance misuse either drugs and or alcohol.

- Accumulative stress e.g. work, relationships, finances

For some it is a combination of all of these. Or for some one cause will lead to another and then another I like to call this the "domino effect".

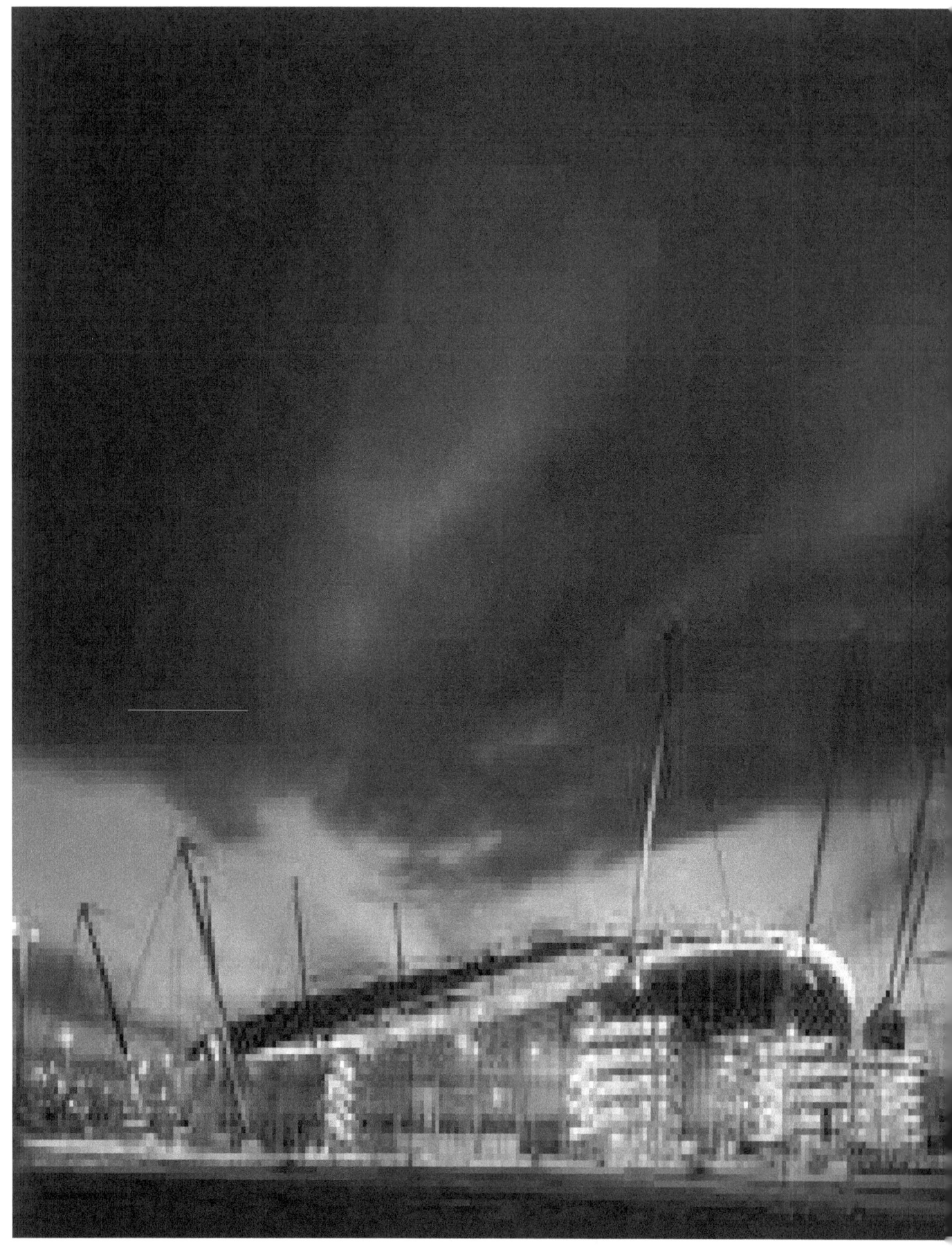

What are the signs and symptoms of poor mental health/illness?

For each person the signs and symptoms are different and below you will find a list of some of these:

- Numbness or tingling anywhere

- Loss of balance

- Double vision or vision problems

- Periods of amnesia

- Co-ordination changes

- Weakness in arms or legs

- Headaches

- Fever

- Nausea/vomiting or diarrhoea/constipation

- Fainting or dizziness, seizures/fits/panic or anxiety attacks

- Changes in appearance and personal hygiene.

- Disturbing thoughts, beliefs and hearing voices.

- Said person becoming distant and isolated.

- Changes in behaviour e.g. different to usual i.e. mild mannered to aggressive.

It's important to remember that all of the above are also side effects that someone may experience from the medications they will be taking to treat there existing issue and it is quite common for some of these to come and go during the time some one is ill.

Again this is not an exhaustive list but some of the most common signs and symptoms and can be experienced singularly or in multiples. If you are being affected by any of these then it is important to contact your G.P. as these can be signs of other illnesses also.

What if I have a diagnosis?

There are many types of diagnosis (often referred to as label) from mild to severe and enduring and amongst some psychiatrists there is a great amount of debate on what is and isn't a mental illness. Some of the most common diagnoses (labels) you will come across are:

- Low Mood – Mild to moderate Depression.

- Clinical Depression.

- Manic Depression/Bi – Polar Disorder.

- Psychotic Depression.

- Schizophrenia

It's important to remember that if you receive one of the above it's not the end but a beginning and that you are not alone.

For most people this is important because it means the end of not knowing what has been wrong and the chance to start putting their lives and relationships back together with all kinds of help and support. Some of which you will find in this book.

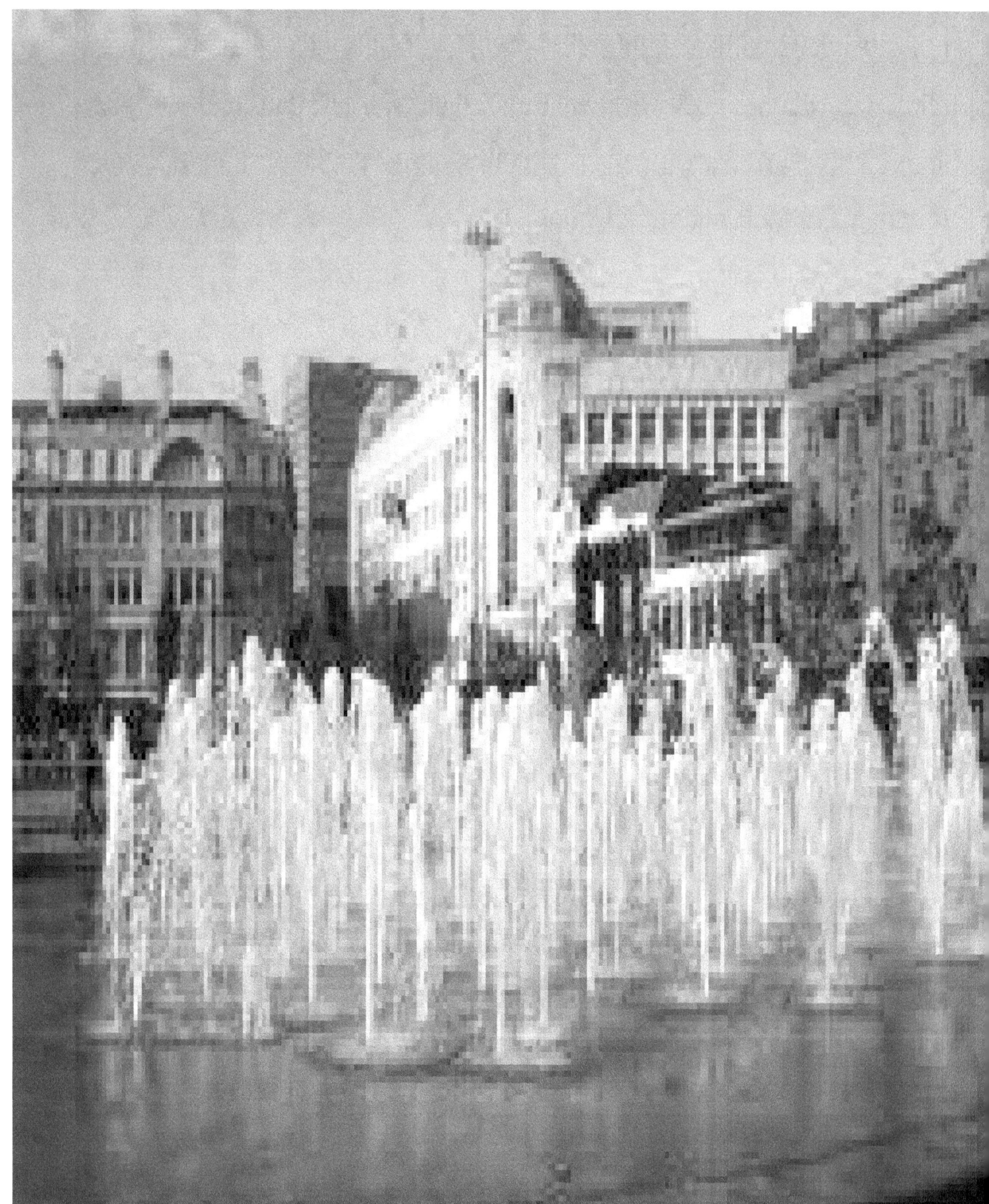

Crisis Support

If you're in an emergency or in crisis and need help then you could try one of the following:

- Contact your G.P.

- Go to your nearest A+E department and ask to speak to a psychiatric liaison nurse.

- Contact NHS Direct.

- Try contacting a helpline where you can talk to someone who can help.

- Or if in doubt call 999 and ask for an ambulance.

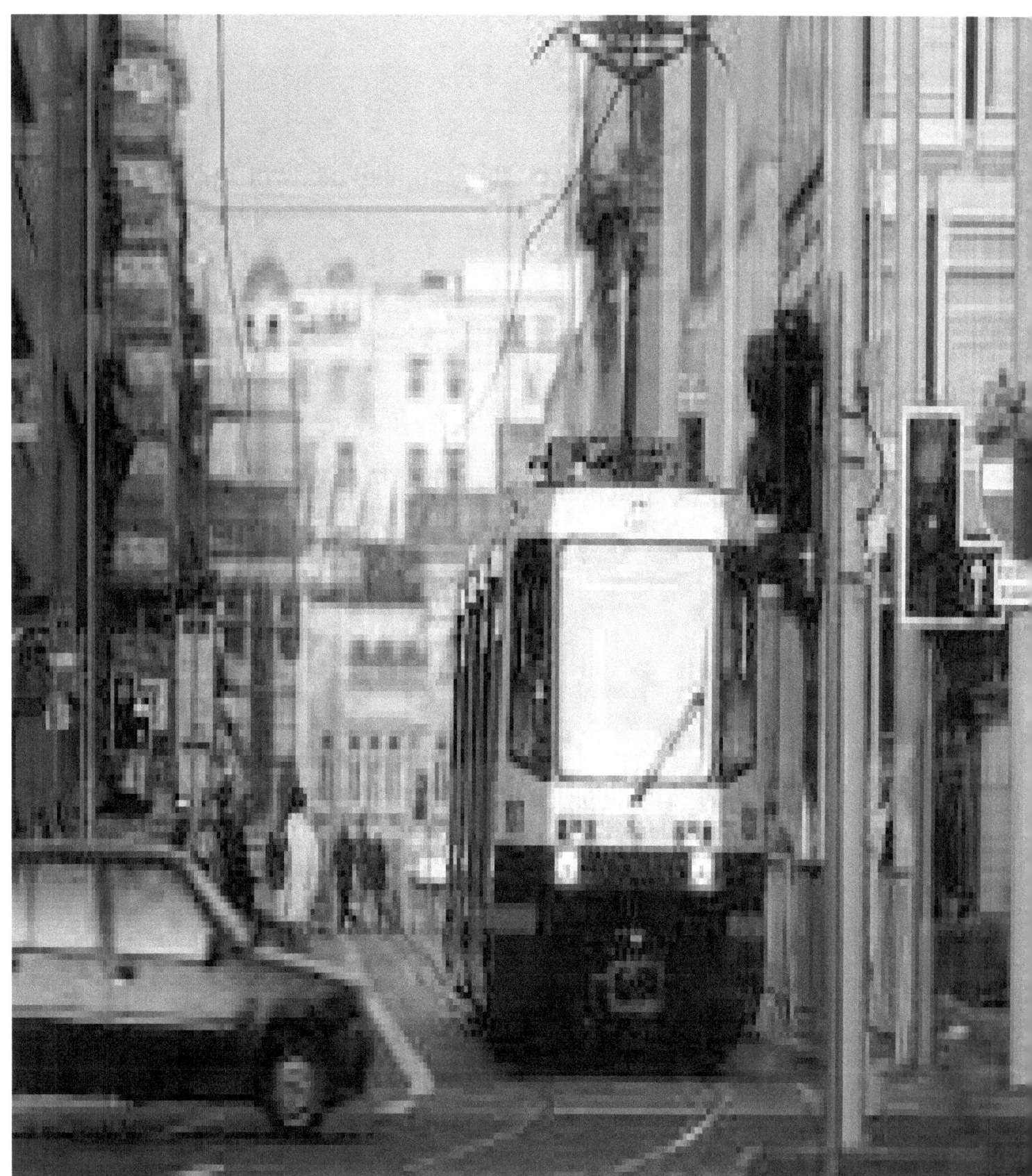

Help lines

Some of the following numbers are for national groups but they will still be able to help and some have more local help they can sign post you to for further help:

- NHS Direct – 0845 4647

- Samaritans – 0845 790 9090/0161 236 8000

- Saneline – 0845 767 8000

- Shelterline – 0808 800 4444

- St Mary's Sexual Assault Helpline – 0161 276 6515

- Victim Support – 0845 303 0900
- Crisis Point – 0161 225 9500

- Ambulance service – 999

If English is not your first language you can contact the Link service on 0161 276 5259 where you will be able to get help in your own language or visit www.recoverymanchester.com where you can find help in our self help section in Arabic, Bengali, Chinese, Somali, Urdu and English.

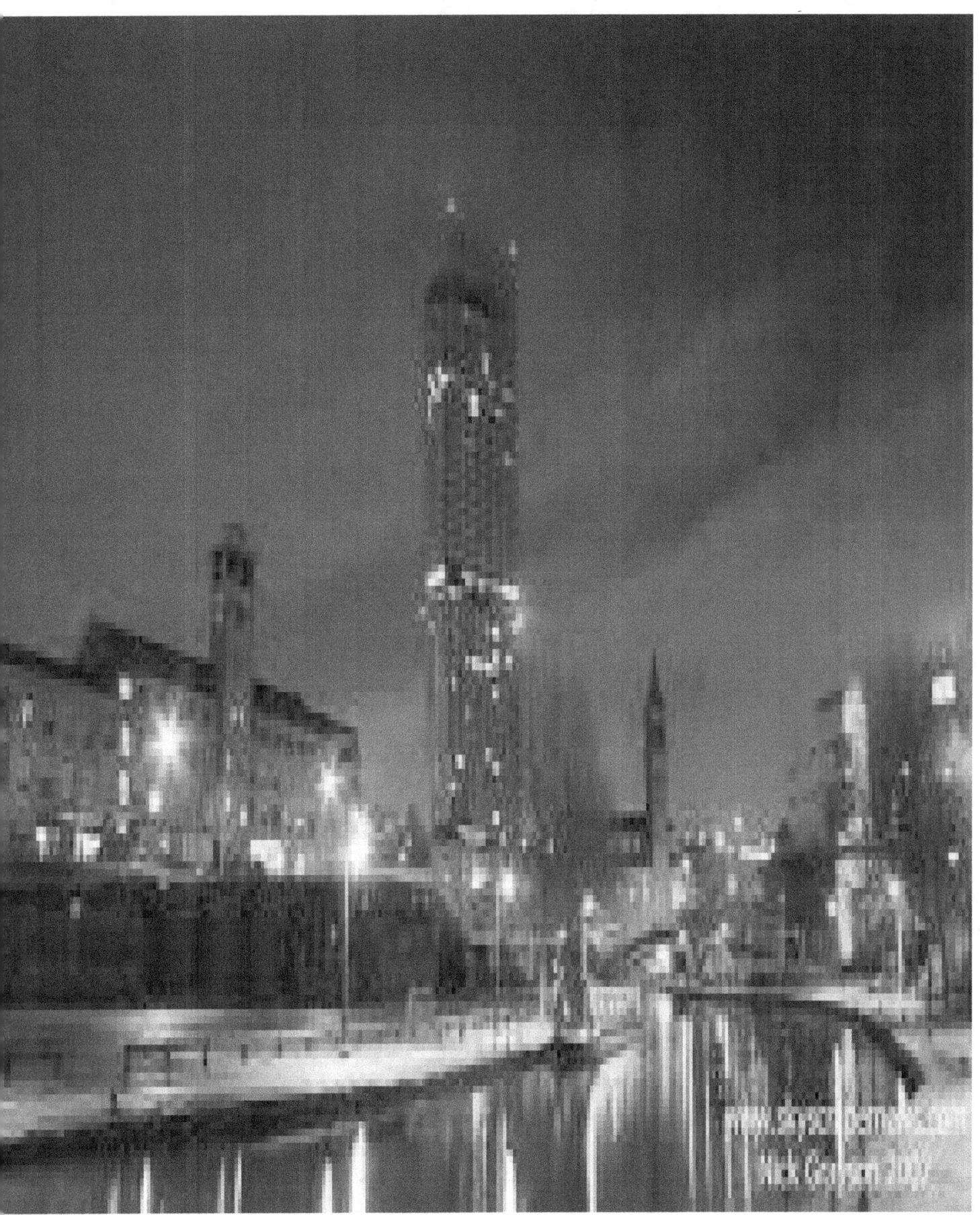

Organisations

Crisis Point

Address: 24 Albert Road
Levenshulme
MANCHESTER
M19 2FP

Contact: 0161 225 9500 Fax: 0161 225 4009

Service: Mental health crisis support centre where people can manage or resolve their crisis and develop strategies to prevent or better manage such crises in the future.

The service can work with people with complex needs and anyone can make a referral, including self referrals.

Services including accommodation (offering stays of up to 10 nights), advice and information, and non-residential one-to-one sessions for up to 6 weeks for people unable or unwilling to use the accommodation service.

Restrictions: Referral 8am - 12 midnight. Mon-Fri 8am - 12pm Sat & Sun 8pm - 12pm

Manchester residents only

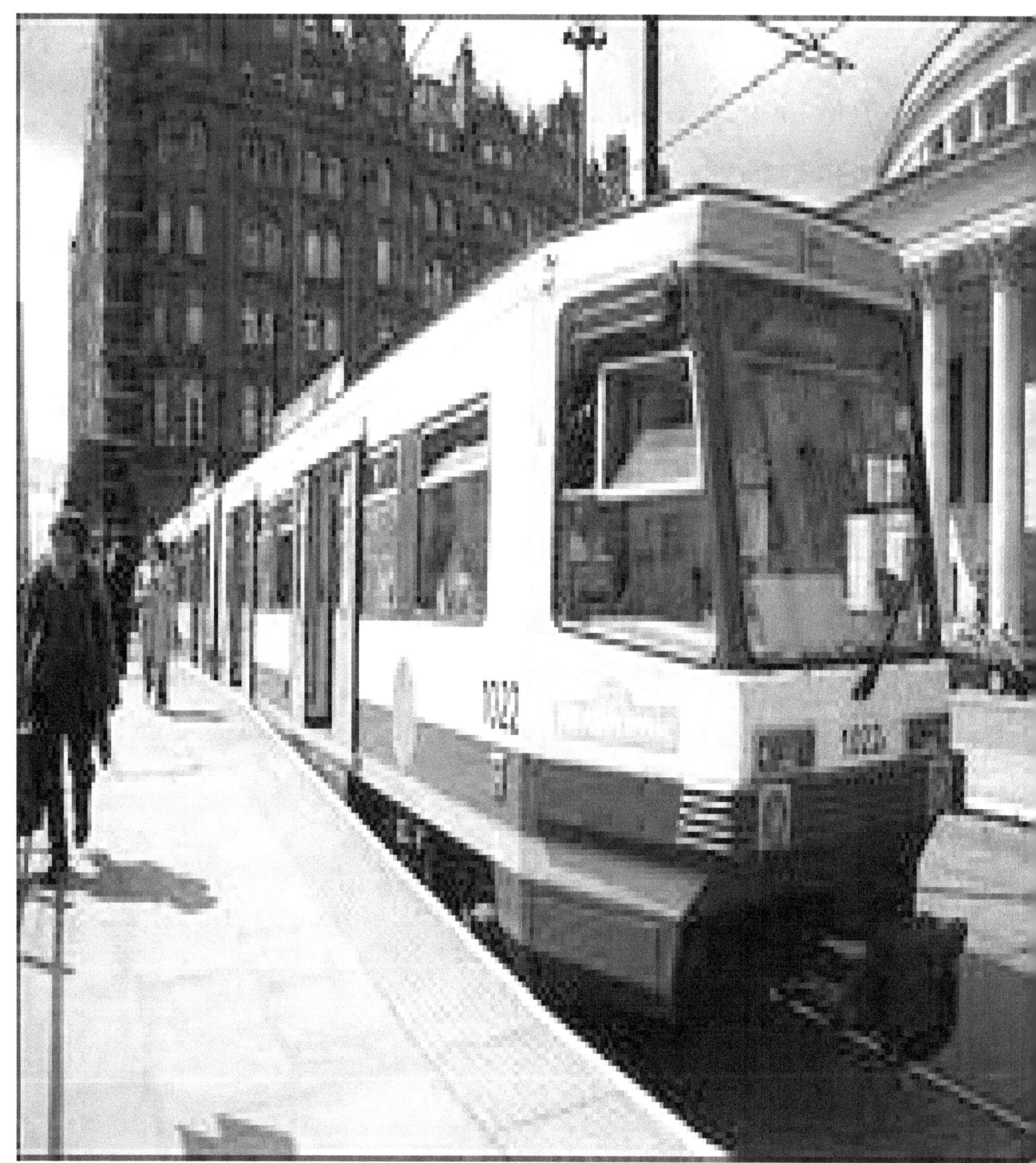

Organisations

The Angel

Address: The Angel Centre
St Philips Place
Salford
Manchester
M3 6FA

Contact: Helen Nelson 07766 550302 Sarah Davidson 07795 306 767

Services: Emergency contraception, Chlamyida screening, Contraceptive implant, fittings and removals, Contraceptive pills and injection

Open Times: wednesday 3pm-6pm

Restrictions: 23s and under

Brook Advisory service

Address: Commonwealth House
      Lever Street
      City Centre
      Manchester
      M1 1FL

Contact: 0161 237 3001 Fax: 0161 236 7047
Email:askbrook@brookmanchester.org.uk
Web Address:www.brook.org.uk

Service: Free confidential sex advice, contraception and counselling for young people. Counselling around any issue, not just sex and relationships.Counselling, Drop In / Day Centre, Employment / Training, Women, Young People

Open: Mon 8am - 1pm 3pm - 7.30pm Tues 12pm - 6.30pm Wed 3pm - 7.30pm Thurs 12pm - 6.30pm Fri 12pm - 4.30pm Sat 11am - 4.30pm. Restrictions: Under 20s only

George House Trust

Address: 77 Ardwick Green North
        MANCHESTER
        M12 6FX

Contact: 0161 274 4499 Fax: 0161 274 3355 email:ght@ght.org.uk
web address:www.ght.org.uk

Services: George House Trust is the HIV charity for the North West,
Emotional & Community Support for people living with HIV
through one-to-one befriending arrangements and support for the
partners, carers and families of people living with HIV. Peer
Support For people living with HIV.

Open: Mon-Fri 9am - 5:30pm

Restrictions: Greater Manchester and North West residents only.

Lesbian and Gay Foundation

Address: 4th Floor
        Princess House
        105 - 107 Princess Street
        MANCHESTER
        M1 6DD

Contact: 0161 330 3030 helpline or office 0161 235 8035. Fax: 0161 235 8036
email:info@lgfoundation.org.uk web address:www.lgfoundation.org.uk

Services: Advocacy, Befriending, Counselling, Drop In / Day Centre, Gay Lesbian & Transgender, Housing Service, Self Help, Women, Young People Helpline operates 6pm - 10pm daily: 0845 330 3030

Open: Office hours 9am – 5pm

Manchester Action on Street Health (MASH)

Address: Unit 15

       Cariocca Business Park

       Miles Platting

       Manchester

       M40 8BB

Contact: 0161 202 2022, 0800 183 0499 email:info@mash.org.uk web address:www.mash.org.uk

Service: MASH offers an outreach service to female sex workers in the greater manchester area. They provide free condoms and lubricants, sexual health advice needle exchange and paraphernalia harm reduction advice/ info a dodgy punter reporting service safety advice and info personal attack alarms assessments/care planning referrals into drug and other services refreshments nightime service

Restriction: females only

Manchester Rape Crisis

Address: P.O Box 336
           M60 2BS

Contact: Helpline 0161 273 4500 BME helpline 0161 273 4514 Fax:
0161 273 4591
email:mrcrasacs@btconnect.com web
address:www.manchesterrapecrisis.co.uk

Service: Counselling, Crisis & Suicide, Ethnic Minorities, Women
Helpline Monday to Friday 10am -4pm; Tuesday, Wednesday and
Thursday 6 - 9pm. 24 hour answering service. Women only service.
Black, minority, ethnic minority helpline on seperate number Mon-
Fri 10am to 4pm (273 4514).

St Mary's Centre - Sexual Assault Referral Centre

Address: St Mary's Centre
St Mary's Hospital
Hathersage Road
MANCHESTER
M13 0JH

Contact: 0161 276 6515 Fax: 0161 276 6691 web address:www.cmmc.nhs.uk/saint-marys/sexual-assault.aspx

Service: Forensic medical examination, Emergency contraception and sexual health screening/advice, Immediate crisis support, Ongoing support through the criminal justice process, access to other healthcare services and community based services, Counselling for clients and their significant others, Training and consultancy services.

Open: Mon-Fri 9am - 5pm 24 hour emergency line: 0161 276 6515

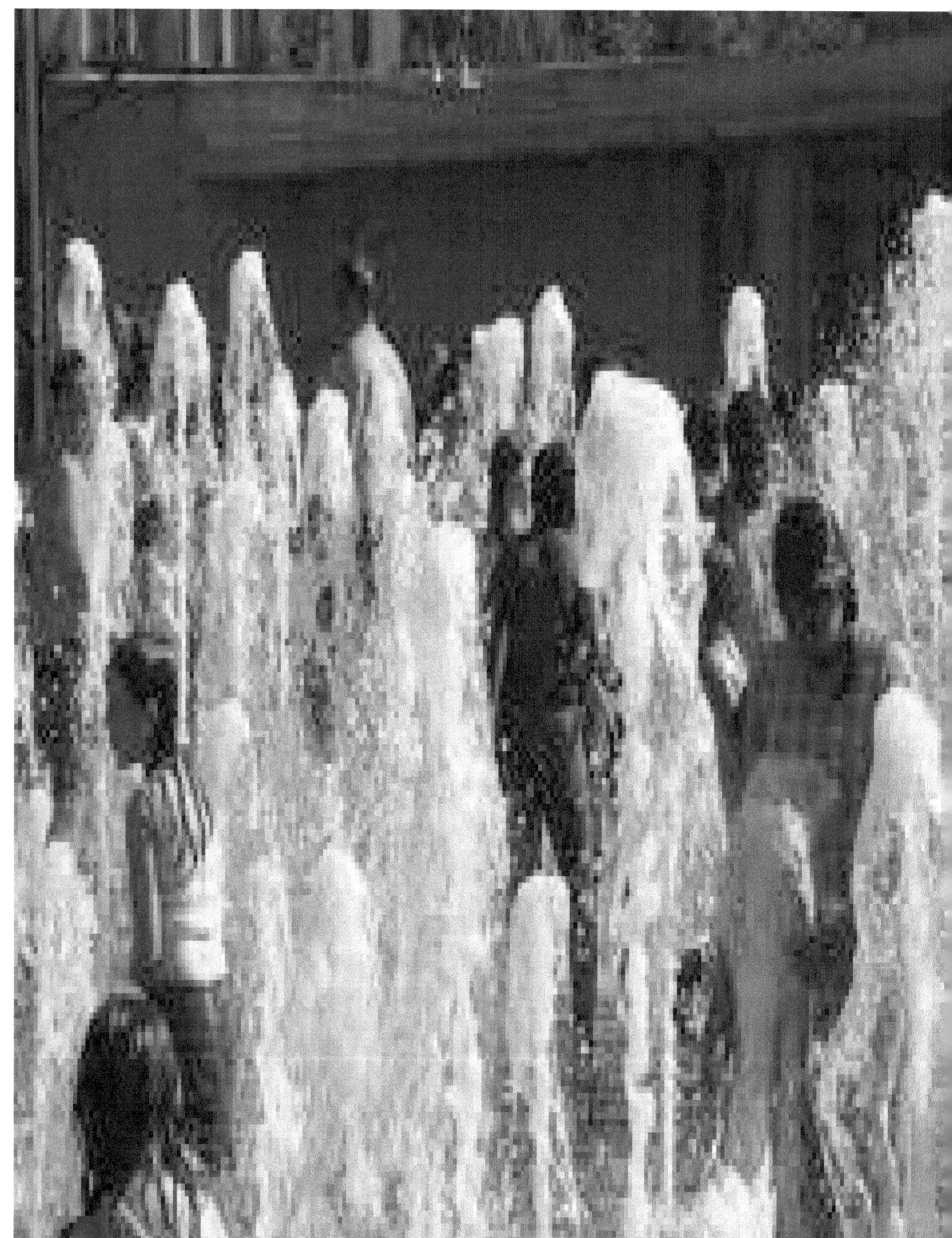

Organisations

42nd Street

Address: 2nd floor Swan Buildings
20 Swan Street
City Centre
MANCHESTER
M4 5JW

Contact: Telephone: 0161 832 0170 Fax: 0161 839 5424 Minicom: 0161 831 7616 Email: theteam@fortysecondstreet.org.uk Web Address: www.fortysecondstreet.org.uk

Services: Counselling, Crisis & Suicide, Depression, Drop In / Day Centre, Ethnic minorities, Gay Lesbian & Transgender, Mental Health Workers, Self Harm, Self Help, Women.

Restrictions: Young People Age 14-25 The Helpline / Referral line is currently staffed: Mon - Fri: 12.30 - 4.30pm

Barnardos After Care Service

Address: Barnardo's Manchester Leaving Care Project

     36 Monton Street

     Moss Side

     Manchester

     M14 4LT

Contact: 0161 226 6722 Fax: 0161 226 5112

Email:frances.bernstein@barnardos.org.uk

www.barnardos.org.uk/leavingcaremanchester

Services: This is a specialist counselling service for Care Leavers at Barnardos Manchester Leaving Care Service. The services provided include - assessment - brief focused therapy, including work on self-harm, bereavement and suicidal feelings - long term therapy of up to 3 years. Open: Mondays to Fridays 9 – 5

Restrictions: Referrals come from within the Leaving Care Service as well as from other professionals and agencies. Self referrals are particularly welcome.

Signpost

Address: St Andrew's Hall
             Brownley Road
             Wythenshawe
             MANCHESTER
             M22 0DW

Contact: 0161 436 5432/436 5433 Fax: 0161 436 1055
email:signpost@pop3.poptel.org.uk web
address:www.signpostadvice.org.uk

Service: Advice, information and support for young people in
Wythenshawe on Benefits / Welfare, Employment / Training,

Open: Mon-Fri 9am - 5pm
Restriction: 14-25 yrs olds in Wythenshawe

YASP

Address: 832 Stockport Rd.
      Levenshulme
      Manchester
      M19 3AW

Contact: 0161 221 3054 Fax: 0161 221 3124 email:info.yasp@harp-project.org web address:www.harp-project.org

Service: Benefits / Welfare, Crisis & Suicide, Drop In / Day Centre, Ethnic Minorities, Housing Service, Mental Health Workers Advice Centre and Drop-in

Open: Mon-Fri 11am - 4:30pm

Restriction: Age 15 – 25

Young Peoples Support Foundation

Address: 52 Oldham Street
MANCHESTER
M4 1LE

Contact: 0161 228 7654 / 5 Fax: 0161 236 5081 web address:www.ypsf.co.uk

Service: Drop In / Day Centre, Employment / Training, Ethnic Minorities, Gay Lesbian & Transgender, Housing Service, User Group

Open: 10am - 12pm and 1pm - 4pm Monday - Friday Closed wednesday afternoons

Restriction: ages 16-25

Young Persons Scheme

Address: 14 Hollinsclough Close
Sharston
Wythenshawe
Manchester
M22 4HS

Contact: 0161 998 9499 Fax: 0161 998 9499
email:yps@creativesupport.org.uk

Services: Benefits / Welfare, Housing Service, Mental Health Workers

Open: 9am – 5pm

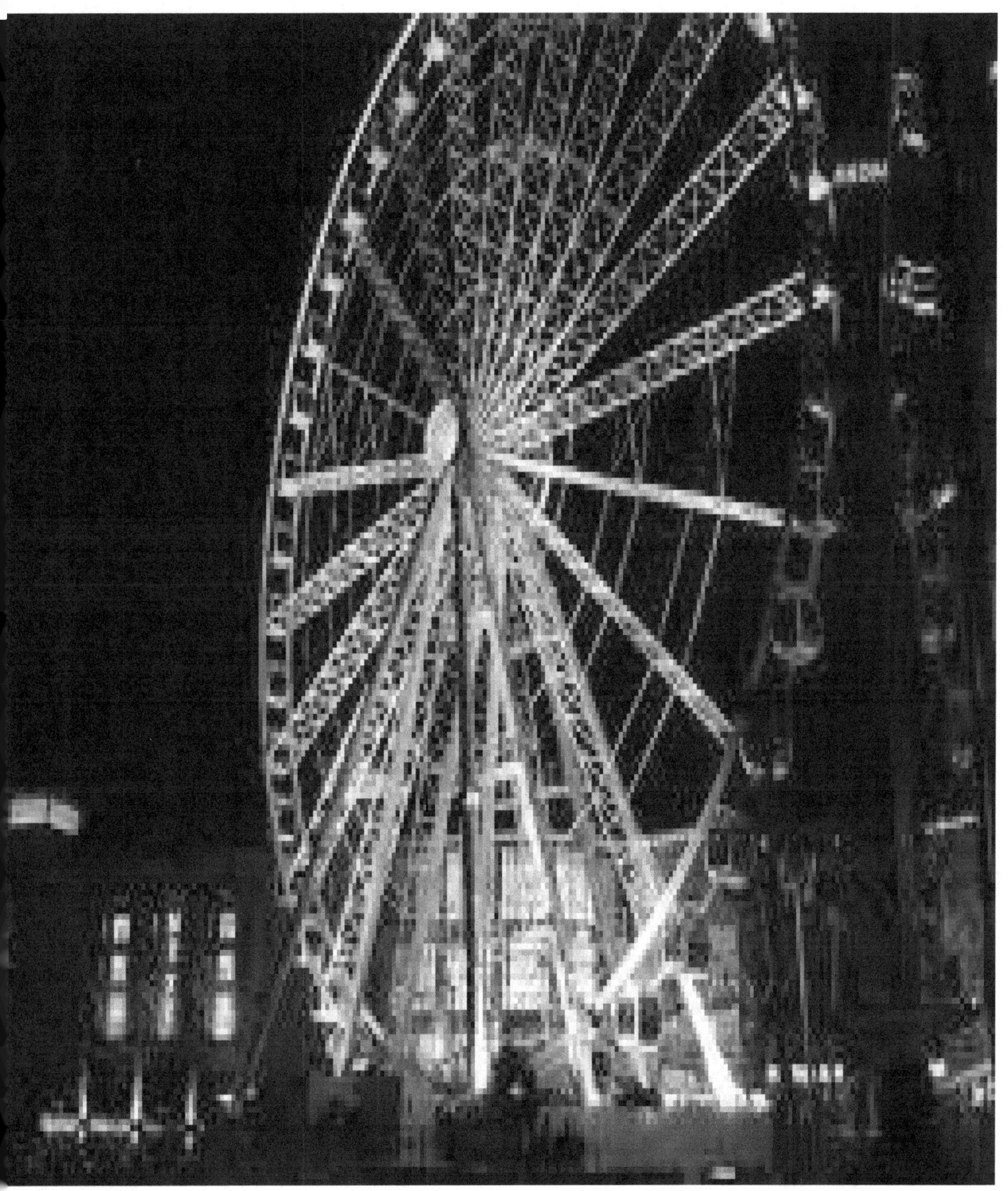

Organisations

A+E Liason Team Central

Address: Manchester Royal Infirmary
        Oxford Road
        Manchester
        M13 9WA

Contact: Telephone: 0161 276 5279
Web Address: www.cmmc.nhs.uk

Services: Crisis & Suicide, Liaison Service 9am - 10pm 7 days a week. A&E department open 24 hours 7 days a week.

Restrictions: Can only be accessed through A&E department

A+E Liason Team North

Address: Delaunays Road
          Crumpsall
          Manchester
          M8 5RB

Contact: Telephone: 0161 720 2560

Service: Crisis & Suicide, Liaison Service 9am - 10pm 7 days a week.
A&E department open 24 hours 7 days a week.

Restrictions: Can only be accessed through A&E department

A+E Liason Team South

Address: Laureate House
          Wythenshawe Hospital
          Southmoor Road
          Wythenshawe
          Manchester
          M23 9LT

Contact: 0161 291 6949 Web Address: www.uhsm.nhs.uk

Services: Crisis & Suicide, Liaison Service 9am - 10pm 7 days a week. A&E department open 24 hours 7 days a week.

Restrictions: Can only be accessed through A&E department

Benchmark

Address: Withington Hospital
      Nell Lane
      Withington
      Manchester
      M20 2LR

Contact: 0161 283 5826 Fax: 0161 283 5826
Email:ask@benchmarkfdab.co.uk
Web Address:www.benchmarkhospitalfurniture.org.uk

Services: Employment / Training, Volunteering

Open: Mon-Fri 9am - 5.30pm

Restrictions: Referral only via CHMT (city wide).

Brian Hore Unit

Address: Withington Community Hospital
         Nell Lane
         West Didsbury
         Manchester
         M20 2LR

Contact: 0161 217 4166 Fax: 0161 217 4936 Web
Address:www.mhsc.nhs.uk

Service: Abstinence based alcohol service offering group and
individual therapy,alcohol & drugs, Drop In / Day Centre, Mental
Health Workers including detox programme
Mon - Fri 9am - 8pm Sat - Sun 9am - 3:30pm

Restriction: Self referral to nursing staff but referral to a
psychiatrist must be from health professional.

Central Manchester Childrens University Hospital

Address: Cobbett House
Manchester Royal Infirmary
Oxford Road
City Centre
MANCHESTER
M13 9WL

Contact: 0161 276 1234 Web Address: www.cmmc.nhs.uk

Service: Hospital and general healthcare services for Central Manchester and specialist services further afield

Open: 24 hours a day.

Restrictions: Central Manchester residents.

Central Manchester Department for clincal health and psychology

Address: Gaskell House
   Swinton Grove
   MANCHESTER
   M13 0EU

Contact: 0161 273 3271 Fax: 0161 273 4825
Email:alison.rainey@mhsc.nhs.uk
Web Address:www.mmhsc.org.uk

Services: Psychological services for adults from Central Manchester

Open: Mon-Fri 9am - 5pm sometimes 4.30pm - Answerphone service availble out of hours

Restrictions: 16-64 years, central Manchester residents only. Referral via GP, Health or Social worker

Central Manchester Primary Care Mental Health Team

Contact: 0161 861 2343 or 861 2344

Service: NHS primary care mental health services, counselling, mental health workers, self help

Open: Monday to Friday 9am-5pm

Restrictions: 16+ G.P referral only

North Manchester Clinical Psychology Service

Address: North Manchester General Hospital
  Delaunays Road
  Crumpsall
  MANCHESTER
  M8 5RL

Contact: 0161 720 2810 Fax: 0161 720 2671

Services: The Clinical Psychology Department sees people experiencing problems in their thoughts, feelings or behaviour with which they are unable to cope e.g. depression, stress, panic, phobias, social confidence problems, addictions, anger control, eating problems and psychosexual problems.

Open: Mon-Fri 9am - 5pm; evening sessions on monday by arrangement.

Restrictions: Referral only by GP's and mental health professionals.

South Manchester Clinical Psychology Service

Address: Laureate House
Wythenshawe Hospital
South Moor Road
Baguley
MANCHESTER
M23 9LT

Contact: 0161 291 6971 Fax: 0161 291 6972

Services: The Clinical Psychology Department sees people experiencing problems in their thoughts, feelings or behaviour with which they are unable to cope e.g. depression, stress, panic, phobias, social confidence problems, addictions, anger control, eating problems and psychosexual problems. Open: 9am - 5pm

Restrictions: Referrals from GPs registered in South Manchester only.

Department of Child and Family Psychiatry

Address: Winnicott Centre
195/7 Hathersage Rd
Victoria Park
MANCHESTER
M13 0JE

Contact: Telephone: 0161 248 9494

Services: Psychiatry and psychotherapy service for children and young people up to the age of 16

Open: .Mon-Fri 9am - 5pm

Restriction: 0-16 year olds referral only

Gaskell House Psychotherapy Centre

Address: Gaskell House Psychotherapy Centre
Swinton Grove
Victoria Park
MANCHESTER
M13 0EU

Contact: 0161 273 2762 Fax: 0161 273 4876
email:admin@psy.cmht.nwest.nhs.uk

Services: Group and individual psychotherapy.

Open: Mon-Fri 9am - 5pm; some evening sessions

Restriction: 16+

Hall Lane Resource Centre

Address: 157-159 Hall Lane
Baguley
Wythenshawe
MANCHESTER
M23 1WD

Contact: 0161 945 7609 Fax:0161 945 7616 web
address:www.mhsc.nhs.uk

Service: A Community Care Mental Health Resource Centre run by Manchester Social Services. The Day Centre offers a Drop-in and various groups for members to share problems, build relationships and join in activities. Members can also receive counselling. Day Centre staff also help run a number of drop-ins in South Manchester and Wythenshawe. Open: Mon-Fri 9am - 4.30pm

Restriction: Mainly South Manchester Residents. Age 16-65 years. Self-referral, via MCC Social Services Dept and other agencies.

Harpurhey Day Centre

Address: 93 Church Lane
Harpurhey
MANCHESTER
M9 5BG

Contact: 0161 205 0118 Fax: 0161 203 4790

Services: Counselling, Drop In / Day Centre, Employment /
Training, Mental Health Workers

Open: Monday to Friday 9am - 4pm

Restriction: Manchester residents aged 16-65yrs

High Elms Drop-in

Address: High Elms
         Upper Park Rd
         Victoria Park
         MANCHESTER
         M14 5RU

Contact: 0161 225 9446 Fax: 0161 225 9446 web address:www.mmhsc.org.uk

Services: High Elms have two community mental health teams working with Psychologists, Social Workers, Occupational Therapists, Nurses, Support Workers and Psychiatrists. They are part of the NHS and referrals are usually via GP or Hospital.

Open: Mon - Thurs: 9am-4pm Fri: 9am-3pm

Restriction:18+

Homeless Mental Health Service

Address: Homeless Mental Health Team
Chest Clinic, 352 Oxford Road
Manchester
M13 9NL

Contact: 0161 273 6908; 272 6973

Service: The small specialist nhs team first gives a mental health assessment for people who are homeless, have a Manchester connection and are not currently seeing a psychiatrist or other mental health service. The team will directly help people with severe or enduring mental health needs, concentrating on short-term intervention. People with other needs will be signposted to the appropriate service. Open: Mon-Fri 9am - 5pm.

Restriction: Staff are generally out of the office but messages can be left. Manchester residents only.

Mainway Enterprises

Address: North Manchester General Hospital
        Delaunays Road
        Crumpsall
        Manchester
        M8 5RB

Contact: 0161 720 2330 Fax: 0161 720 2996
email:info@mainway.org.uk
web address:www.mainway.org.uk

Service: Mainway Enterprises is a service offering supported employment opportunities to people with severe and enduring mental health needs. The service offers a range of work placements based around a structured day and the development of work skills.

Manchester Assertive Outreach Team

Address: PO Box 201

        M21 8WR

Contact: 0845 0068 999 Fax: 0845 0063 999 email:info.mao@harp-project.org

www.harp-project.org/projects/project_ngage_index.php

Service: This is an intensive support for people with severe mental illness and complex needs who are not engaging with services, including those with a dual diagnosis of mental health needs and substance misuse. The assertive outreach workers provide practical support towards social inclusion with medical back-up including specialist treatment where necessary.

Open: Mon-Fri 8am - 8pm Sat & Sun 10 - 6pm
Restriction: Manchester residents only

Manchester Community Alcohol Team

Address: c/o Beswick District Office
        1 Campion Walk
        MANCHESTER
        M11 3RS

Contact: 0161 223 9641 Fax: 0161 230 7811 web address:www.manchestercat.org

Service: Alcohol & Drugs, Counselling

Open: Mon-Fri 9am - 4pm (24hr answerphone)

Restriction: Manchester residents only. Do not see people under 16 years of age.

Manchester Mental Health and Social Care Trust

Address: Chorlton House
70 Manchester Road
Chorlton-cum-Hardy
MANCHESTER
M21 9UN

Contact: 0161 882 1000 Fax: 0161 882 1001
email:www.mhsc.nhs.uk/contact.aspx?p=435 web
address:www.mhsc.nhs.uk

Service: Crisis & Suicide, Employment / Training, Hospital Service,
Mental Health Workers, Older People

Open: Mon-Fri 9am - 5pm

Restriction: Services are provided to people registered with a GP in
Manchester only

Manchester Mental Health Single Point of Access (SPA)

Address: Edale House
       Manchester Royal Infimary
       Oxford Road
       Manchester
       M13 9WL

Contact: 0161 276 6155 Fax: 0161 276 6154 web address:www.mhsc.nhs.uk

Service: Hospital Service, Mental Health Workers

Open: Mon-Fri 8am - 6pm

Manchester Primary Care Trust PALS Service

Contact: 0161 219 9451

www.manchesterpct.nhs.uk/yourviewscount/pals/palsquery.aspx

Service: The Patient Advice & Liaison Service (PALS) service can answer any questions you have as a patient, relative, carer, friend of a patient or any other member of the public about the services provided by Manchester Primary Care Trust. The service can listen to your concerns and suggestions, provide on-the-spot information on NHS services and help sort out problems quickly on your behalf.

Open: Monday - Friday 9am - 5pm

North Manchester Primary Care Mental Health Team

Contact: 0161 237 0017

web address: www.manchesterpct.nhs.uk

Service: Manchester Primary Care Mental Health Services offer short term support to residents, aged 16 and older, who are registered with a GP and have common mental health problems and/or associated social problems such as anxiety and panic, phobias, depression, bereavement difficulties, obsessions, compulsions and stress related problems.

PEARL

Address: Edale House

Manchester Royal Infirmary

Oxford Road

Manchester

M13 9WL

Contact: 0161 901 1477 web address:www.mhsc.nhs.uk

Service: Crisis & Suicide, Hospital Service

Open: 24 hours a day, seven days a week

PRAMMBS (Psychiatric Referral, Assessment and Management of Mothers and Babies Service)Andersen Ward

Address: Laureate House
        Wythenshawe Hospital
        South Moor Road
        Baguley
        Manchester
        M23 9LT

Contact: 0161 291 6829 Fax: 0161 291 6821 web address:www.mhsc.nhs.uk

Service: Regional service for women with babies of less than one year old who have moderate to severe mental health problems.

Open: 24 hours a day.
Restriction: The service will only take referrals from mental health professionals.

SAFE Team

Address: Rawnsley Building
        Manchester Royal Infirmary
        Oxford Road
        MANCHESTER
        M13 9WL

Contact: 0161 276 8865 Fax: 0161 276 8872 web address:www.mhsc.nhs.uk

Service: SAFE is short for Self Harm, Assessment, Follow-up and Engagement

South Manchester Primary Care Mental Health Team

Address: Forum Health
Simons Way
Wythenshaw
M22 5RX

Contact: 0161 435 3698

Service: Counselling, Mental Health Workers, Self Help

Restriction: Strictly G.P referral

Victoria Park Day Centre

Address: Victoria Park Centre
70 Daisy Bank Road
Victoria Park
MANCHESTER
M14 5QN

Contact: 0161 224 1308 Fax: 0161 256 2740
email:mike.grierson@manchester.gov.uk

Service: Drop In / Day Centre, Self Help, User Group, Volunteering, Women

Open: Mon 9am - 4pm Tue 9am - 4pm Wed 9am - 7pm Thu & Fri 9am - 4pm

Restrictions: Only open to people on enhanced CPA

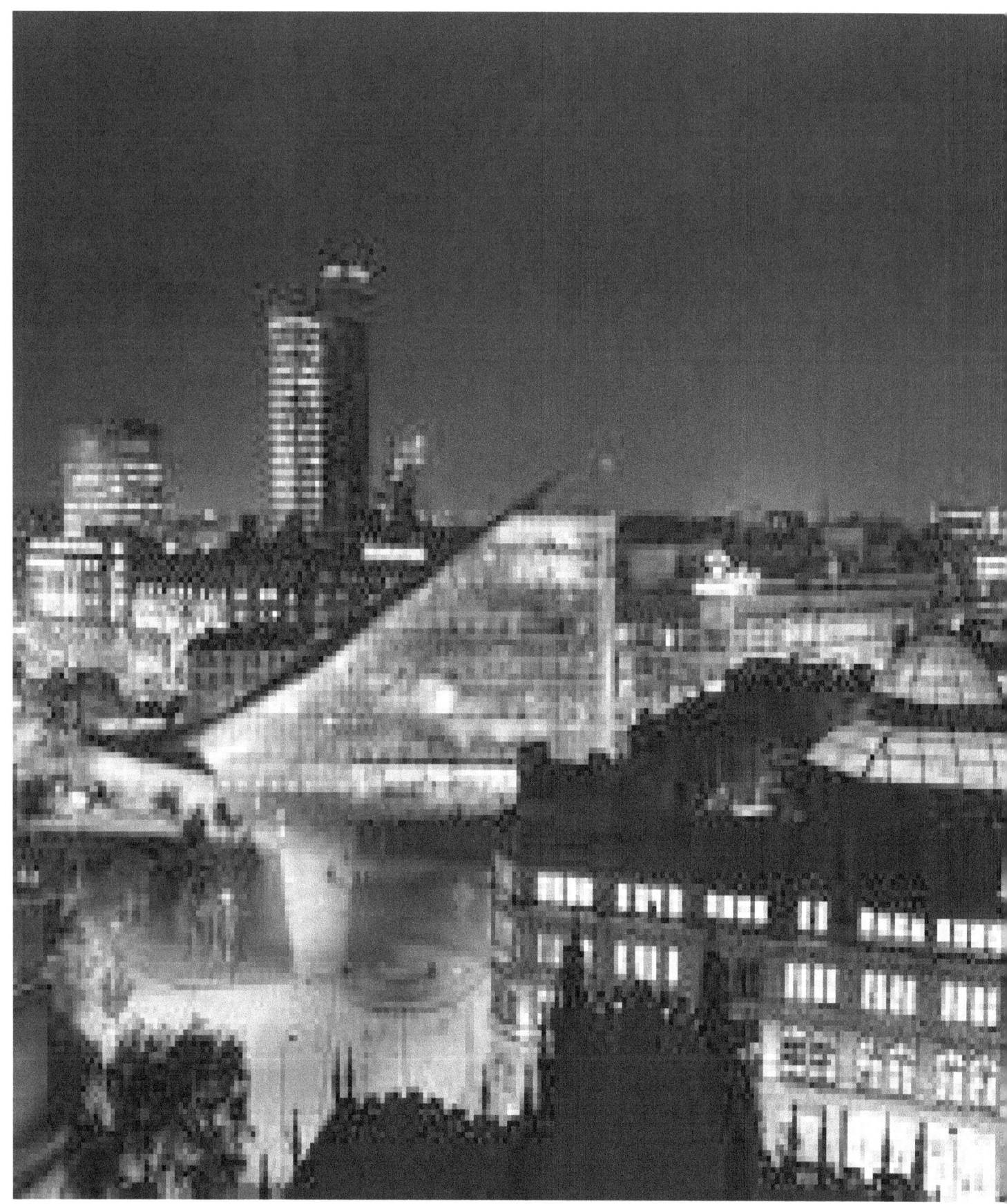

Organisation

A4E Connect

Address: WorkSuite G, Ground Floor
125 Portland Sreet
Manchester
M1 4QD

Contact: 0161 237 3405 email: kmurray@a4e.co.uk Web Address:
www.a4econnecttowork.co.uk

Services: CV and interview preparation, Confidence building,
Up to 52 weeks in work support, A discretionary back to work fund.

Open: Monday till Friday 9-5

Restrictions: Must be on benefits to access service

Break Through UK

Address: Business Employment Venture Centre
Aked Close
Ardwick
MANCHESTER
M12 4AN

Contact: 0161 273 5412 Fax: 0161 274 4053
Email:admin@breakthrough-uk.co.uk
Web Address:www.breakthrough-uk.com

Services: Disability, Employment / Training

Open: Mon-Fri 8.30am - 5pm

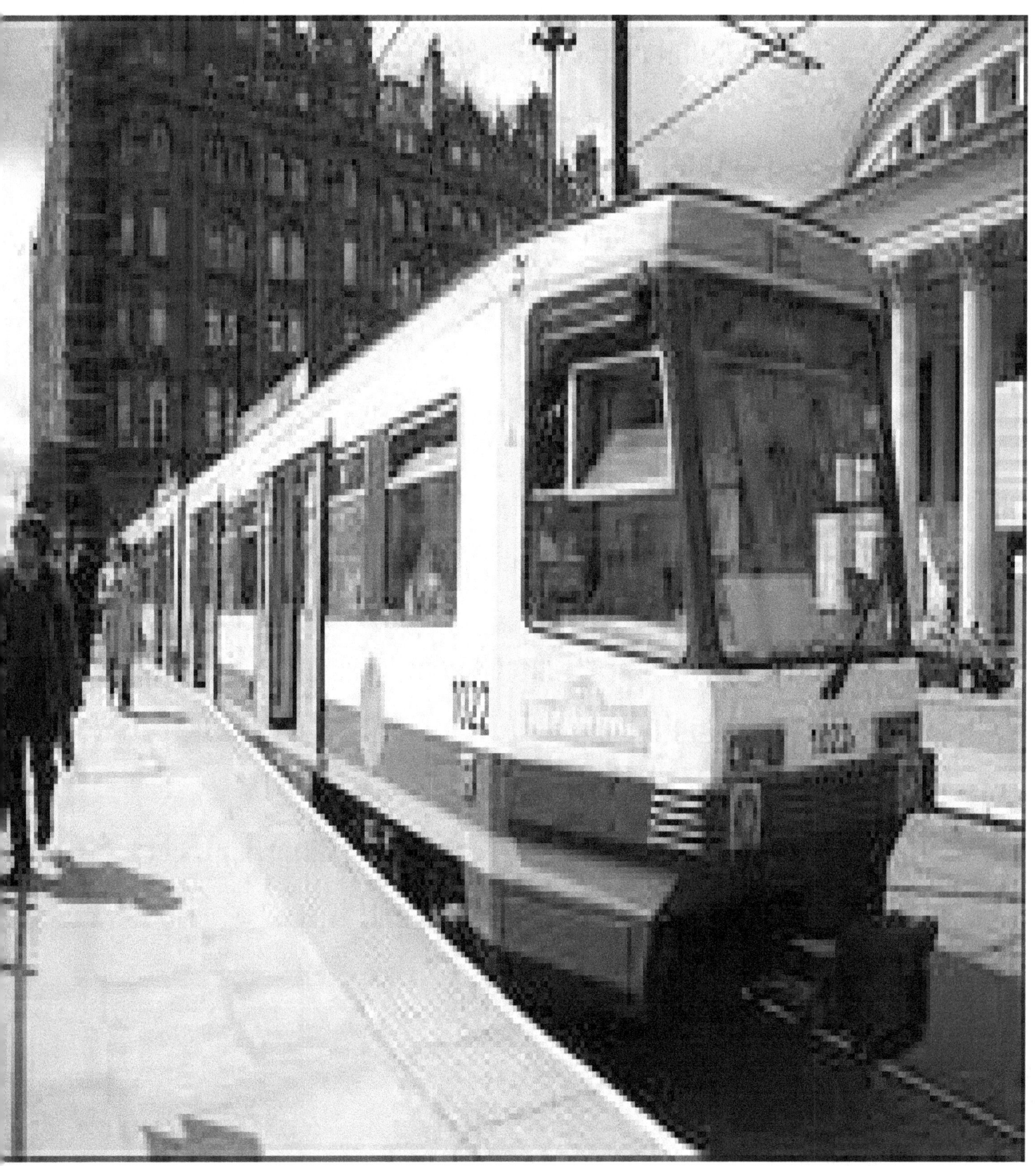

Advice and Community Resource Centre

Address: 59 Withington Road
               Whalley Range
               MANCHESTER
               M16 7EX

Contact: Telephone: 0161 226 7015 Fax: 0161 226 7524 email: family-advice-c@mcr1.poptel.org.uk

Services: Benefits / Welfare, Employment / Training, Housing Service, Legal, Volunteering,

Open: Advice sessions: Tue & Wed 10am - 12:30pm Thursday 1:30pm - 4pm Office: Mon-Fri 9:30am - 5pm

Cheetham Hill Advice Service

Address: 1 Morrowfield Avenue
       Cheetham Hill
       MANCHESTER
       M8 9AR

Contact: 0161 740 8999 Fax: 0161 720 9231
Email:office@cheethamadvice.org.uk
Web Address:www.cheethamhilladvicecentre.org.uk

Services: Advocacy, Benefits / Welfare, Ethnic Minorities, Housing Service, Legal, Volunteering,

Open: Advice Sessions: by appointment only Mon-Thu. drop-in: Tue from 10am

Restrictions: Residents of Cheetham Hill and Crumpsall area (M8 postcode)

Gaddum Centre

Address: Gaddum House
6 Great Jackson Street
City Centre
MANCHESTER
M15 4AX

Contact: 0161 834 6069 Fax: 0161 839 8574
web address: www.gaddumcentre.co.uk/source/home.htm

Services: The Information Line in Manchester is available on 0161 839 0421 and can answer questions about social and health care needs, people's rights under Community Care, Disability and Children's legislation.

Other services provided include:-

- Advocacy Services
- Other Related Independent Reportage Services

- Children and Families Bereavement Service
- Social Work Counselling in Primary Care
- Staff Care Service
- Older Persons Visiting Service
- Trust Administration
- Training & Education Mon-Fri 9am - 4:30pm

Information Line Mon-Fri 1:15pm - 4:30pm.

Restrictions: Manchester residents only

Greater Manchester Pay and Employment Rights Advice Service

Address: 4th Floor, Swan Buildings
   20 Swan Street
   City Centre
   MANCHESTER
   M4 5JW

Contact: 0161 839 3888 advice line office 0161 839 3882 Fax: 0161 839 3883
email:info@gmemploymentrights.org.uk
web address:www.gmlpu.org.uk

Service: Telephone advice on pay and employment rights.

Open: Mon-Fri: 10am - 4pm

Restrictions: Greater Manchester area residents only

HARP (Health Advocacy Resource Project)

Address: Zion Centre
339 Stretford Road
Hulme
MANCHESTER
M15 4ZY

Contact: 0161 226 9907 Fax: 0161 232 9970 email:info@harp-project.org web address: www.harp-project.org

Services: Advocacy, Benefits / Welfare, Drop In / Day Centre, Employment / Training, Housing Service, Mental Health Workers, Volunteering

Open: Mon-Fri 9am - 5pm

Independent Complaints Advocacy Service

Address: Barnett House

53 Fountain Street

Manchester

M2 2AN

Contact: 0845 120 3732 or 0161 247 8649

email:icas@carersfederation.co.uk

Web Address: www.carersfederation.co.uk

Services: They provide a self help pack, involve an iterpreter if need be, meet you in a place where you feel comfortable if unable to come to the office. The advocates can help you write letters to the right people, prepare you for meetings, give you the opportunity to speak to someone who is independent of the NHS, answer questions to help you make decisions, act on your direction rather than wishes of others.

Open: Mon - Fri 9am - 5pm

Independent Employment Advocacy Project

Address: Breakthrough UK Ltd

       B.E.V.C

       Aked Close

       Ardwick

       MANCHESTER

       M12 4AN

Contact: 0161 273 5412 Fax: 0161 274 4053

email:admin@breakthrough-uk.co.uk

web address: www.breakthrough-uk.com

Services: Breakthrough UK Ltd aims to remove barriers to employment and independent living for disabled people.

Open: Mon-Fri 9am - 5pm

Restrictions: Greater Manchester residents Only

Manchester Advice Centre

Address: P.O. Box 536
        Town Hall Extension
        MANCHESTER
        M60 2AF

Contact: 0161 234 5678 Fax: 0161 234 3320
email:advice@manchester.gov.uk
web address:www.manchester.gov.uk

Service: Advocacy, Benefits / Welfare, Housing Service, Legal
telephone advice Mon-Fri 10am - 4pm

Drop-in Mon,Tues,Thurs,Fri 9am – 4.30pm Weds 10am - 4-30pm

Manchester Advice Mental Health Welfare Rights Service

Address: Harpurhey Ditrict Office 8 Moston Lane
       Harpurhey Manchester
       M9 4DP

Contact: 0161 205 7321 Fax: 0161 205 8921
email:city.council@manchester.gov.uk
www.manchester.gov.uk/advice/welfare/mhealth.htm

Service: Advocacy, Benefits / Welfare, Employment / Training,
Housing Service, legal advice, by appointment

Open: 9am - 5pm

Restriction: Residents of the City of Manchester (and Manchester
City Council Employees) only. Location within the city not
important if can get to venues.

Manchester Carers Centre

Address: Beswick House
Beswick Row
MANCHESTER
M4 4PR

Contact: 0161 835 2995 Fax: 0161 835 3845
email:admin@manchestercarers.org.uk
web address:www.carers.org/manchester

Service: Advocacy, Carers / Family, Drop In / Day Centre, Self Help,
Volunteering

Open: Mon - Fri 9:30am - 4:30pm Carersline: 835 4090

Restriction: For adult carers living or caring for someone in the City
of Manchester

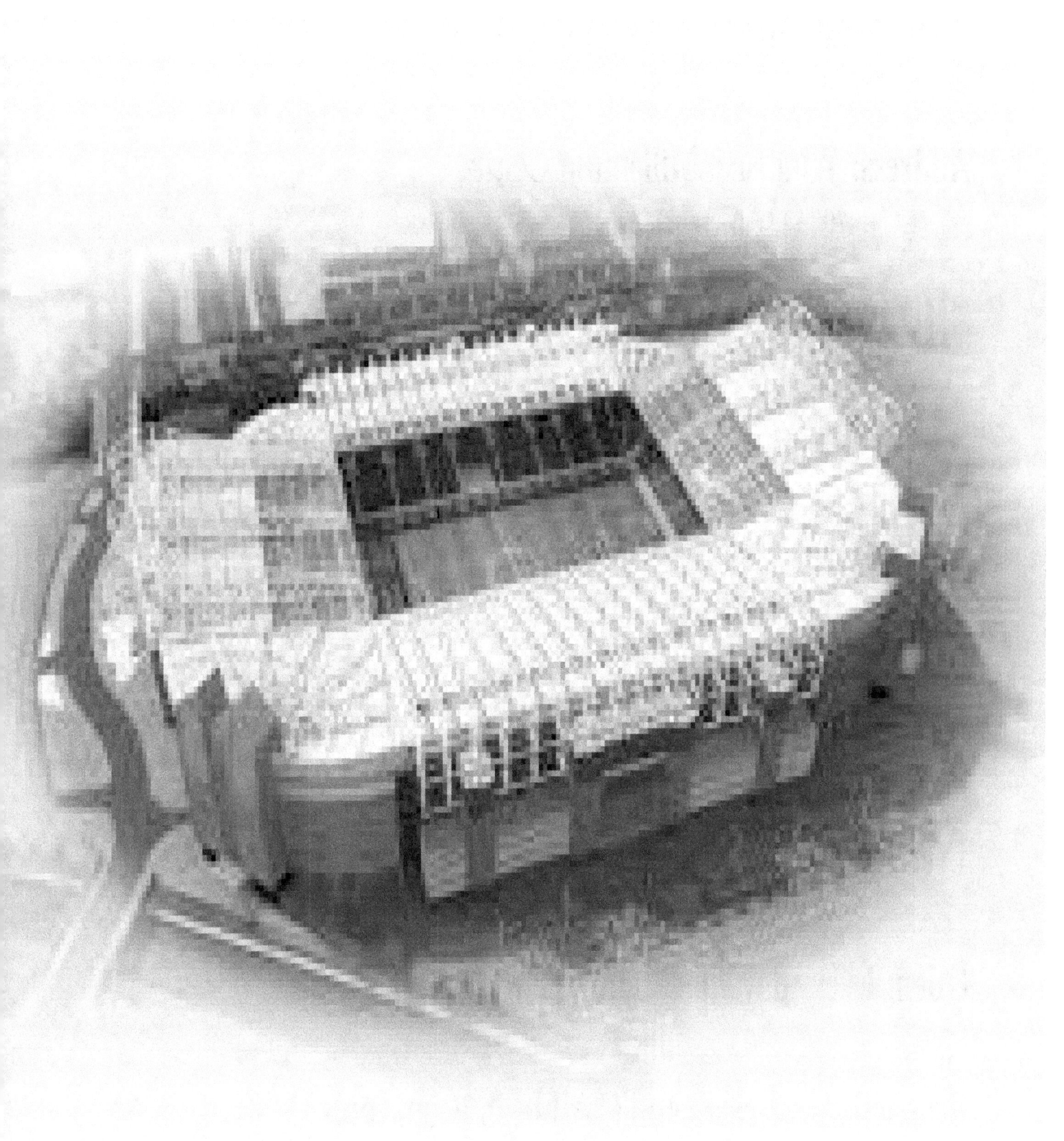

Afro Carabean Mental Health Services

Address: Windrush Millenium Centre
70 Alexandra Road
Mosside
Manchester
M16 7WD

Contact: Telephone: 0161 226 9562/ 4829 Fax: 0161 226-7947 email: admin@cmhs-blackmentalhealth.org.uk

Services: Advocacy, Benefits / Welfare, Carers / Family, Counselling, Drop In / Day Centre, Employment / Training, Ethnic Minorities, User Group, Volunteering

Open: Every day 9am - 5pm

Restrictions: African and Caribbean people only.

ANANNA Womens Bangladeshi Organisation

Address: 360 Dickenson Road
   Longsight
   MANCHESTER
   M13 0NG

Contact: 0161 257 3867 Fax: 0161 257 3867
email:anannamcr@aol.com

Services: Mental Health Helpline 257 2122 open 9:00am - 3:00pm.

Mental Health and health workers giving practical advice and support.

- English as a Second Language (ESOL) class Tuesday 9:30 - 11:30am

- Yoga classes Tuesday 1:30 - 2:30pm

- Mother and toddler group Tuesday 1:30 - 3:00pm

- Young women's group Friday 1:00 - 3:00pm

- Keep fit class Monday 9:30 - 11:00am Wednesday 1:00 - 2:30pm

- Well women drop-in 1.00 - 3.00pm

- Classroom Assistant Wednesday 10:00am - 12:30pm, 10 week course Friday 10:00am - 12:30pm

- Beauty session Friday 1:00 - 2:00pm

Restrictions: Bangladeshi women but women from other racial groups welcome. Languages Bengali and Urdu

Asian Young Girls and womens group

Address: Longsight Youth Centre
        422 Stockport Rd
        Longsight
        MANCHESTER
        M12 4EX

Contact: 0161 273 2946 Fax: 0161 273 1998

Services: Befriending, Counselling, Ethnic Minorities, Self Help, Volunteering, Women, Young People Ring or call in 12:30pm - 2pm to make appointment. Answering machine available at other times.

Restrictions: Young Asian women only

Irish Community Care

Address: 289 Cheetham Hill Road
         Cheetham
         Manchester
         M19 3PZ

Contact: 0161 205 9105 Fax: 0161 203 4627
email:mcr.irish@zetnet.co.uk
web address: www.iccmanchester.org.uk

Service: Advice, information and support for Irish and wider community in Manchester. Projects for Irish Travellers, young people, elderly. Advice and casework on welfare benefits, housing, ID, health issues, training, and returning to live in Ireland. Men's over 40s group. Over 50s Social and Craft group. Outreach sessions in Levenshulme

Open: Mon-Fri 10am-4pm

Linkworkers Advice Service

Address: P.O. Box 536
        Town Hall Extension
        MANCHESTER
        M60 2AF

Contact: 0161 234 5600 Fax: 0161 234 3320 web
address:www.manchester.gov.uk/advice/linkwork

Service: Linkworkers service is a free and confidential advice service. It produces practical help and information on a variety of issues including, housing, benefits and Council Services.

They hold advice sessions at Community Centres throughout the City, as well as offering a home visit service to people who are housebound.

Call the following numbers for further details:-

- 0161 272 7826 Arabic
- 0161 272 7825 African
- 0161 272 7853 African Caribbean
- 0161 272 7826 Arabic
- 0161 272 7823 Bangladeshi / Sylheti
- 0161 740 9468 Bosnian
- 0161 272 7822 Cantonese
- 0161 720 7574 Gujarati / Kutchi / Hindi
- 0161 272 7824 Somaili
- 0161 272 7827 Urdu / Punjabi
- 0161 720 8463 Vietnamese

Weekly drop-in advice sessions.

Restriction: Manchester residents only

Longsight and Moss Side Community Project

Address: 95A Princess Road
Moss Side
M14 4TH

Contact: 0161 226 4632 Fax: 0161 226 4632
email:imcp@btconnect.com

Services: Befriending, Counselling, Drop In / Day Centre, Employment / Training, Ethnic Minorities, Older People, Volunteering, Women

Open: Mon-Fri 9am - 5pm; drop-ins Mon 10-3 Thurs 1-3

Restriction: Asian women with mental health needs in Manchester. 50+

Manchester Refugee Support Network

Address: St James Centre
        95A Princess Road
        Moss Side
        Manchester
        M14 4TH

Contact: 0161 232 7420 web address:www.mrsn.org.uk

Service: Advocacy, Benefits / Welfare, Ethnic Minorities

Open: Mon - Fri 10-5

Pakistani Resource Centre

Address: 1 Great Marlborough Street
         MANCHESTER
         M1 5NJ

Contact: 0161 237 1125 Fax: 0161 237 9556 email:info@pakistani-resource.org.uk
web address:www.pakistani-resource.org.uk

Service: Advocacy, Benefits / Welfare, Carers / Family, Counselling, Drop In / Day Centre, Employment / Training, Ethnic Minorities, Housing Service

Open: Mon-Fri 9am - 4:30pm

Restriction: Members of the south Asian communities

Refugee Action – Manchester

Address: 23-37 Edge St
MANCHESTER
M4 1HW

Contact: 0800 917 2719 free client advice line Fax: 0161 831 5420
web address:www.refugee-action.org.uk/manchester

Service: Gives practical support and advice to refugees & newly
arrived asylum seekers and promotes their rights in the UK and
abroad.

Drop in Mon and Thurs from 9.30 am. Appointments only at other
times.

Restrictions: 16+

Sahara Project

Address: Cornbrook Enterprise Centere
        70 Quenby Street
        Hulme
        Manchester
        M15 4HW

Contact: 0161 835 3393 Fax: 0161 835 2055
email:jennifer@blackhealthagencey.org.uk
web address:www.blackhealthagencey.org.uk

Service: Advocacy, Alcohol & Drugs, Benefits / Welfare, Crisis &
Suicide, Depression, Ethnic Minorities, Learning Disability, Manic
Depression / Bipolar, Mental Health Workers, Older People,
Schizophrenia, Self Harm, Volunteering, Young People

Open: Office hours, usually home visits arranged

Restriction: Residents of North Manchester.

Wai Yin - Kwan Wai Project

Address: 1st Floor
61 Mosley Street
Manchester
M2 3HZ

Contact: 0161 237 5908 Fax: 0161 228 3096
email:info@waiyin.org.uk
web address:www.waiyin.org.uk

Service: Carers / Family, Ethnic Minorities, Mental Health Workers,
Self Help

Open: Mon-Thu, Sat & Sun 10am - 6pm

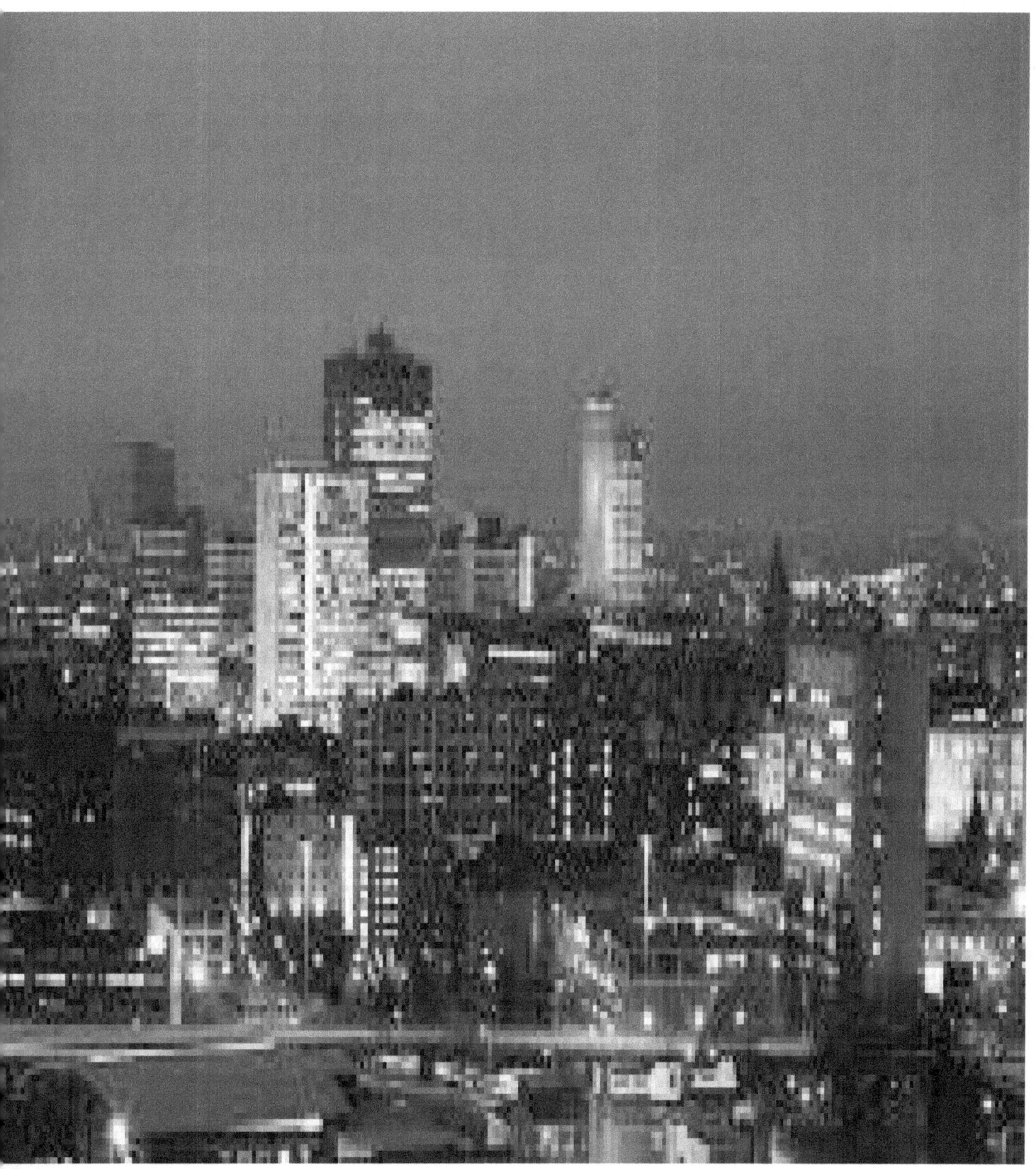

Age Concern Manchester

Address: 20 Swan Buildings
Swan Street
Manchester
M4 5JW

Contact: Telephone: 0161 833 3944 Fax: 0161 833 3945 email:
enquiries@silverservice.org.uk Web Address:
www.silverservice.org.uk

Services: Advocacy, Benefits / Welfare, Carers / Family, Counselling,
Drop In / Day Centre, Ethnic Minorities, Older People, Volunteering

Open: Mon-Fri 9am - 5pm

Age Concern (National)

Address: Astral House
1268 London Road
LONDON
SW16 4ER

Contact: Telephone: 0800 00 99 66 Fax: 0208 765 7211 email: ace@ace.org.uk www.ageconcern.org.uk

Services: Campaigner on ageing issues and the major provider of local care services for all older people. Benefits / Welfare, Drop In / Day Centre, Older People, Self Help

Helpline is open 8am - 7pm, seven days a week. Mon-Fri 9am - 5pm.

Restrictions: Services are for the over 60's only

Altzimers Society Manchester

Address: Phoenix Mill
5-6 Piercy Street
Ancoats
MANCHESTER
M4 7HY

Contact: 0161 203 6434 Fax: 0161 205 8738
email:manchester@alzheimers.org.uk
Web Address: www.alzheimers.org.uk

Services: Home from Hospital Befriending Service (contact:
emma.sleith@alzheimers.org.uk) Dementia Outreach Service
(debbie.smith@alzheimers.org.uk) Carers Breaks at Home Service
(jenny.merron@alzheimers.org.uk)

Open: Mon-Fri 9am - 5pm.
Restrictions: Carers of people with dementia in Manchester

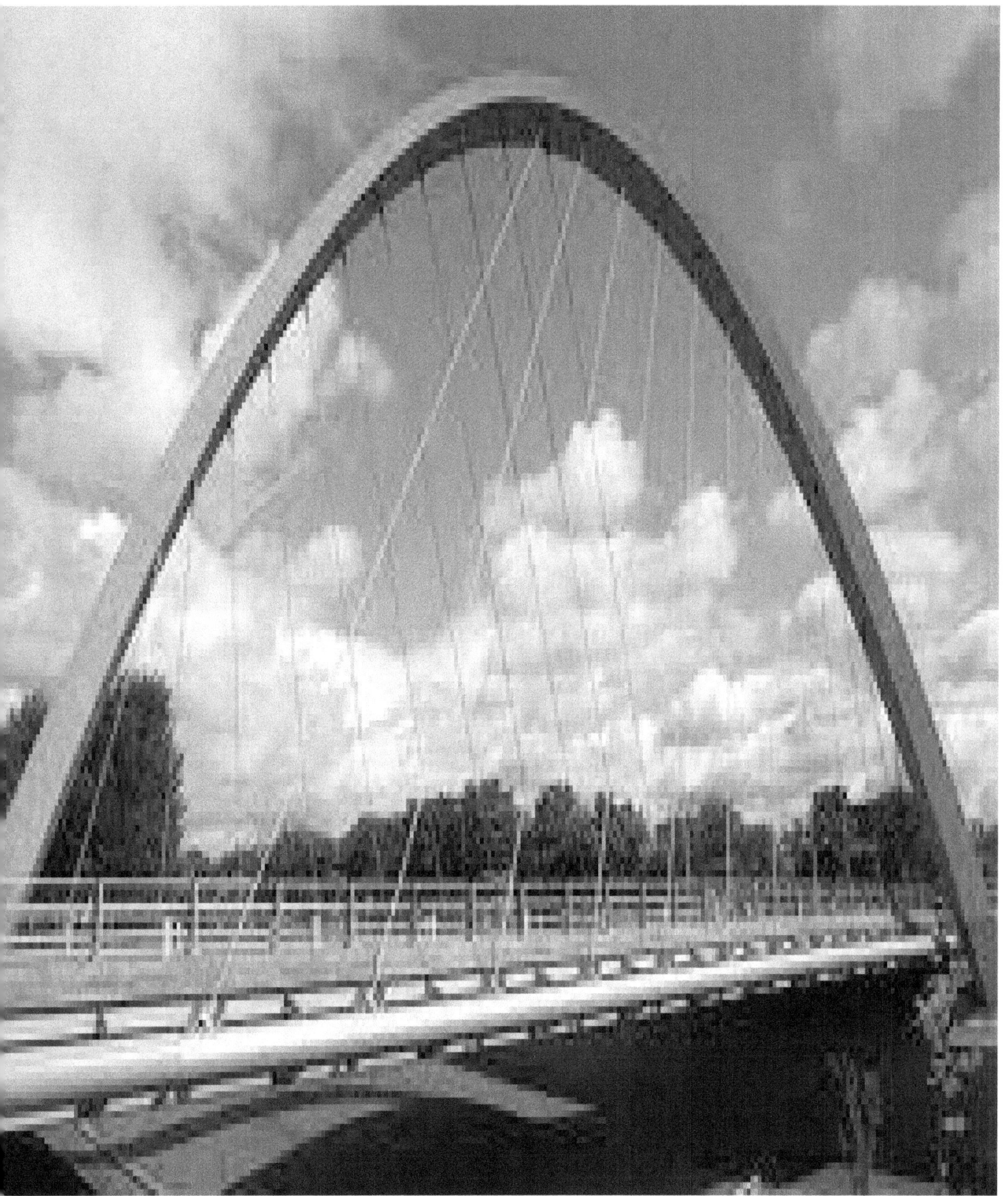

ADS

Address: 29a Ardwick Green North
        Ardwick
        MANCHESTER
        M12 6FZ

Contact: 0161 272 8844 Fax: 0161 272 8899
email:ads@alcoholanddrugservices.org.uk
Web Address: www.alcoholanddrugservices.org

Services: Community Alcohol Services; Day Care Services; Criminal Justice Services; Primary Health Care Services; Residential Services; Training Services; Black and Ethnic Services.

Open: Monday 9am-8pm Tues,Weds,Fri 9am-5pm Thurs 9am-8pm Sat 10am-2pm

Restrictions: There are no counselling services from this branch

DASH

Address: The Zion Centre
339 Stretford Road
Hulme
MANCHESTER
M15 4ZY

Contact: 0161 226 0202 Fax: 0161 226 5989

Service: Alcohol & Drugs, Carers / Family, Counselling, Drop In / Day Centre, Employment / Training, Ethnic Minorities, Gay Lesbian & Transgender, User Group, Volunteering

Open: Monday 1pm-5pm Tuesday 10am-7pm Wednesday 10am-5pm Thursday 10am-7pm Friday 10am-5pm

Restriction:18+ only.

Frank Cohen Support Group

Address: 223 Moston Lane
Moston
MANCHESTER
M9 4HE

Contact: 0161 205 7508

Services: Frank Cohen Support Group provides support and activities for alcoholics and ex-drinkers.

The Drop-in is open 7 days a week.

There is a counselling service on Wednesdays from 6.00p.m-9.00p.m. Referral: self or via doctors

Drop-in: Mon-Sat 9am - 12.30pm;

Restriction: Strictly No alcohol allowed

Lifeline Project – Manchester

Address: 101-103 Oldham Street
City Centre
MANCHESTER
M4 1LW

Contact: 0161 834 7160 Fax: 0161 834 5903
email:webeditor@lifeline.org.uk
web address:www.lifeline.org.uk

Services: Alcohol & Drugs, Counselling, Self Help, Young People

Open: Mon-Thurs 9:30am - 8pm; Fri 9:30am - 5pm

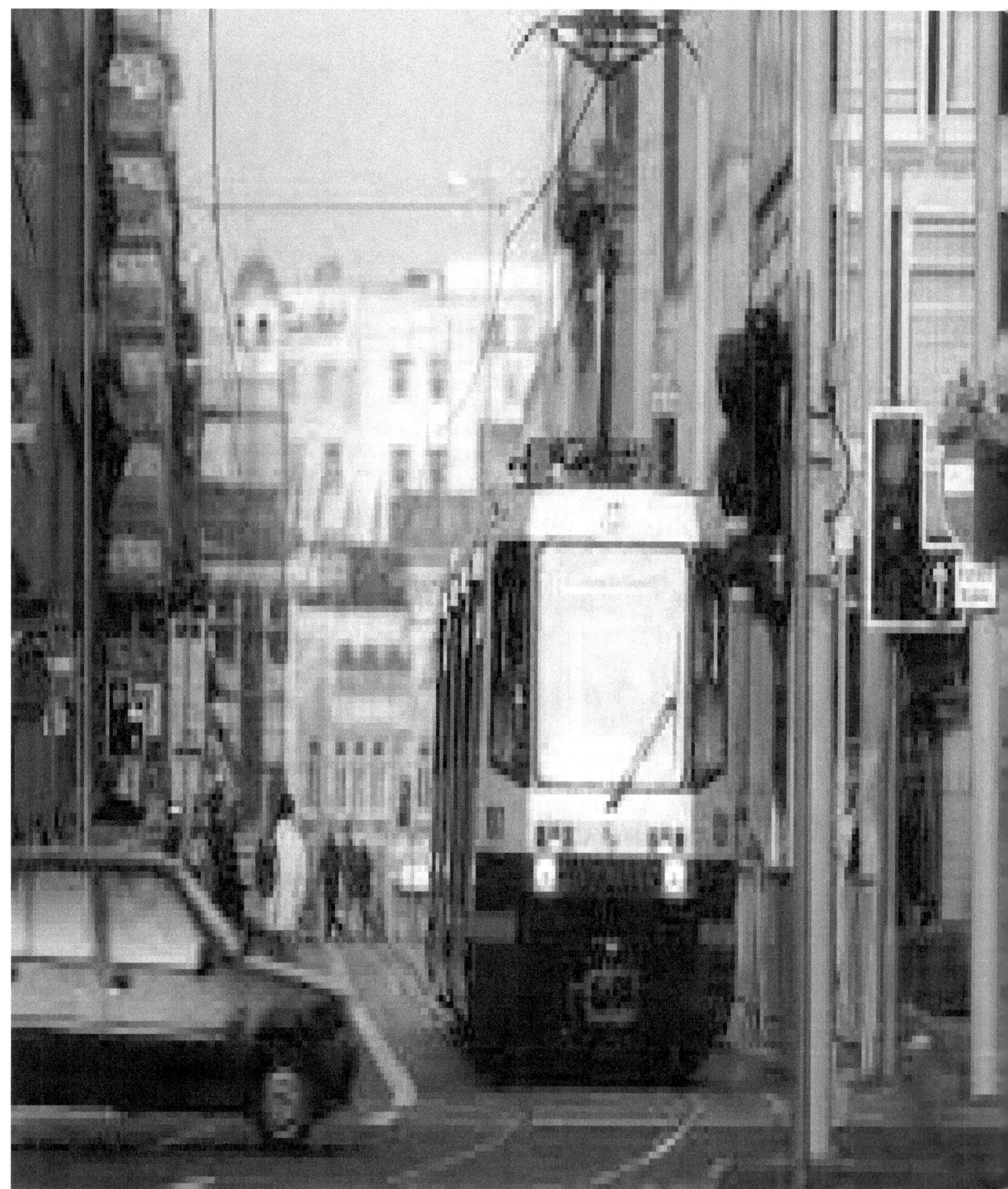

Alternatives to Violence Project

Address: 6 Mount Street (Bootle Street entrance)
  City Centre
  Manchester
  M2 5NS

Contact: 0161 832 3660 email: avpgmr@yahoo.co.uk Web Address: www.avpbritain.org.uk

Services: A national network of volunteers running workshops for anyone who wants to find ways of resolving conflict without resorting to violence.

Workshops in Greater Manchester are open to everyone and usually take place over one weekend. Fees are modest and there are concessions for people on low incomes.

DV-LAP

Contact: Telephone: 0161 881 0911

Service: Legal advocacy, support and advice for women experiencing domestic violence

Open: Mon-Fri 10am - 4pm An answerphone service is available at other times and your call will be returned.

Restriction: For women only

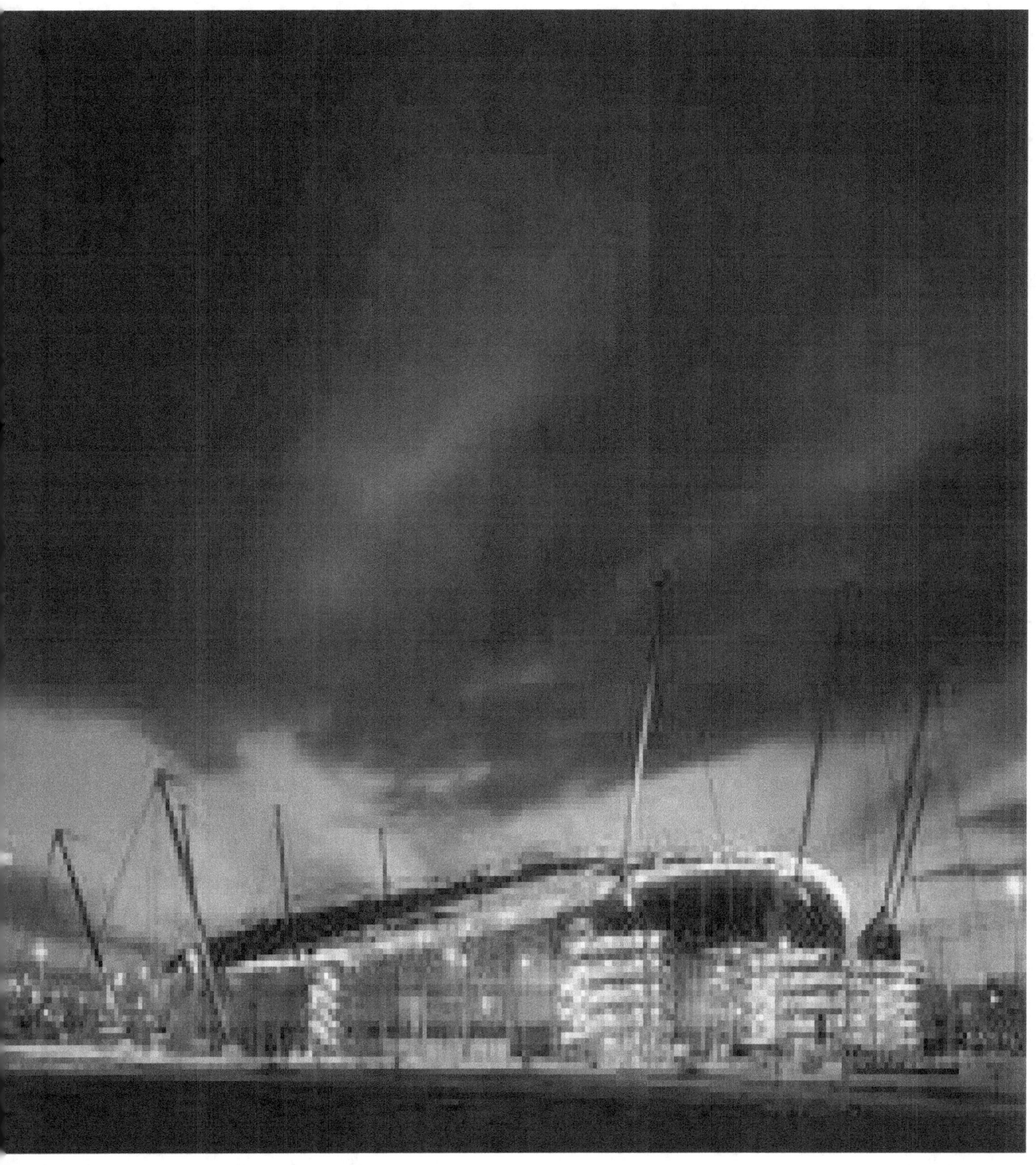

Ann Lee Centre

Address: 12 Hilton St
         Manchester
         M1 1JF

Contact: 0845 1203711 email:info@annleecentre.org.uk
Web Address: www.annleecentre.org.uk

Services: Mental Health Workers, Self Help, User Group,
Volunteering.

Open: Monday to Fiday 10am-4pm

Restrictions: 18+ only

Aspirations

Address: 1114 Chester Road
           Stretford
           MANCHESTER
           M32 0HL

Contact: 0161 866 8485 Fax: 0161 789 2628
Email: aspirations@asgma.org.uk

Services: Supports young people with Asperger Syndrome in Greater Manchester via Drop In / Day Centre, Learning Disability, Self Help, Young People

Open: Mon-Fri 9am - 5pm

Restrictions: For ages 10 – 25

Eating Disorders Self-help Group

Address: The Zion Centre
339 Stretford Road
Hulme
MANCHESTER
M15 4ZY

Contact: Telephone: 0870 770 0740
email:info@self-helpservices.org.uk
web address:www.self-helpservices.org.uk

Services: The group is aimed at anyone affected by any kind of eating disorder. Members can meet, have a drink, and talk to others who have been in a similar situation, in a safe, caring and suportive environment. Information on disorders is available.

Open: Tuesdays 6pm-8pm/Restrictions: The group is aimed at both males and females, 18 years plus. 16 and 17 year olds are welcome to attend with an over-18 parent, sibling, friend or care giver etc.

Hearing Voices Network

Address: 79 Lever Street.
Manchester
M1 1FL

Contact: 0845 122 8641
email:info@hearing-voices.org
web address:www.hearing-voices.org

Services: Schizophrenia, Self Help, User Group

Open: Office Mon-Fri 10am - 4pm.

Helpline Tue 1-4pm

Kath Locke Centre

Address: 123 Moss Lane East
Hulme
MANCHESTER
M15 5DD

Contact: 0161 455 0211 Fax: 0161 455 0213
email:kathlocke@diverseresources.org.uk
web address: www.kathlocke.org.uk

Services: Anxiety, Drop In / Day Centre, Ethnic Minorities, Learning Disability, Mental Health Workers, Self Help, User Group, Volunteering

Open: Mon-Fri 9am - 5pm

Restriction: Residents of Manchester Only

Manchester Carers Forum

Address: Swan Buildings
   20 Swan Street
   Manchester
   M4 5JW

Contact: 0161 629 9859 Fax: 0161 629 9756
email:info@manchestercarersforum.org.uk
web address:www.manchestercarersforum.org.uk

Service: Befriending, Carers / Family, Self Help, User Group

Open: Mon-Fri 9am - 5pm

Restriction: For carers in the Manchester area.

Mood Swings Network

Address: 23 New Mount Street
City Centre
MANCHESTER
M4 4DE

Contact: Helpline 0845 123 6050 Fax: 0161 953 4105
email:helpline@moodswings.org.uk

Service: Carers / Family, Depression, Employment / Training, Manic Depression / Bipolar, Older People, Self Help, User Group, Volunteering, Young People

Helpline open 10am - 4pm for people with mood disorders, their carers, other mental health organisations

Samaritans - Manchester and Salford Branch

Address: 72-74 Oxford Street
       City Centre
       MANCHESTER
       M1 5NH

Contact: 0161 236 8000 email:jo@samaritans.org
web address:www.manchester@samaritans.org

Service: Assistance of persons who are suicidal, despairing or in distress in Manchester Befriending, Counselling, Crisis & Suicide, Depression, Drop In / Day Centre, Volunteering

Open: Phone 24 hours 7 days a week. Visit 9am - 8:30pm

Self Help Services

Address: Zion Centre
        339 Stretford Road
        Hulme
        MANCHESTER
        M15 4ZY

Contact: 0844 477 9971 Fax: 0161 226 7727
email:info@selfhelpservices.org.uk
web address:www.selfhelpservices.org.uk/

Service: Alcohol & Drugs, Anxiety, Carers / Family, Counselling, Depression, Ethnic Minorities, Gay Lesbian & Transgender, Manic Depression / Bipolar, Self Harm, Self Help, Volunteering, Women

Enquiries 9:30am - 5:30pm Groups meet at various times - phone for details.

Restrictions: Self referral and GP referral. 16+

South Manchester User Group

Address: Laurent House
        Wythenshawe Hospital
        Wythenshawe
        MANCHESTER
        M23 1WD

Contact: 0161 291 6860 Fax: 0161 291 6861 email:sm.ug@uku.co.uk

Service: South Manchester User group have offices in Hall Lane
Resource Centre. It is a strictly user-driven service, offering drop-
ins, befriending and advocacy.

Hall Lane drop-in Sun 12 - 3.30

Mobile number availble 24hrs 07921995479 Current and former
users of psychiatric services

St Luke's Church & Neighbourhood Centre Drop-in

Address: St. Luke's Drop-in
1 Guide Post Square
Longsight
M13 9EA

Contact: 0161 273 1538 email:rogerhoward@btconnect.com

Service: Counselling, Drop In / Day Centre, Mental Health Workers, Self Help, Volunteering, Women Various times for each activity

The Roby Church

Address: Dickenson Road
 Longsight
 MANCHESTER
 M13 0NG

Contact: 0161 257 2653 Fax: 0161 257 2653
email:roby@mcr13.freeserve.co.uk
web address:www.theroby.org.uk

Services: Counselling, Drop In / Day Centre, Ethnic Minorities, Self Help, User Group, Womens Drop-in: Thu 10am - 1pm Counselling available Mon - Fri 9.30 am - 5 pm; plus evenings possible.

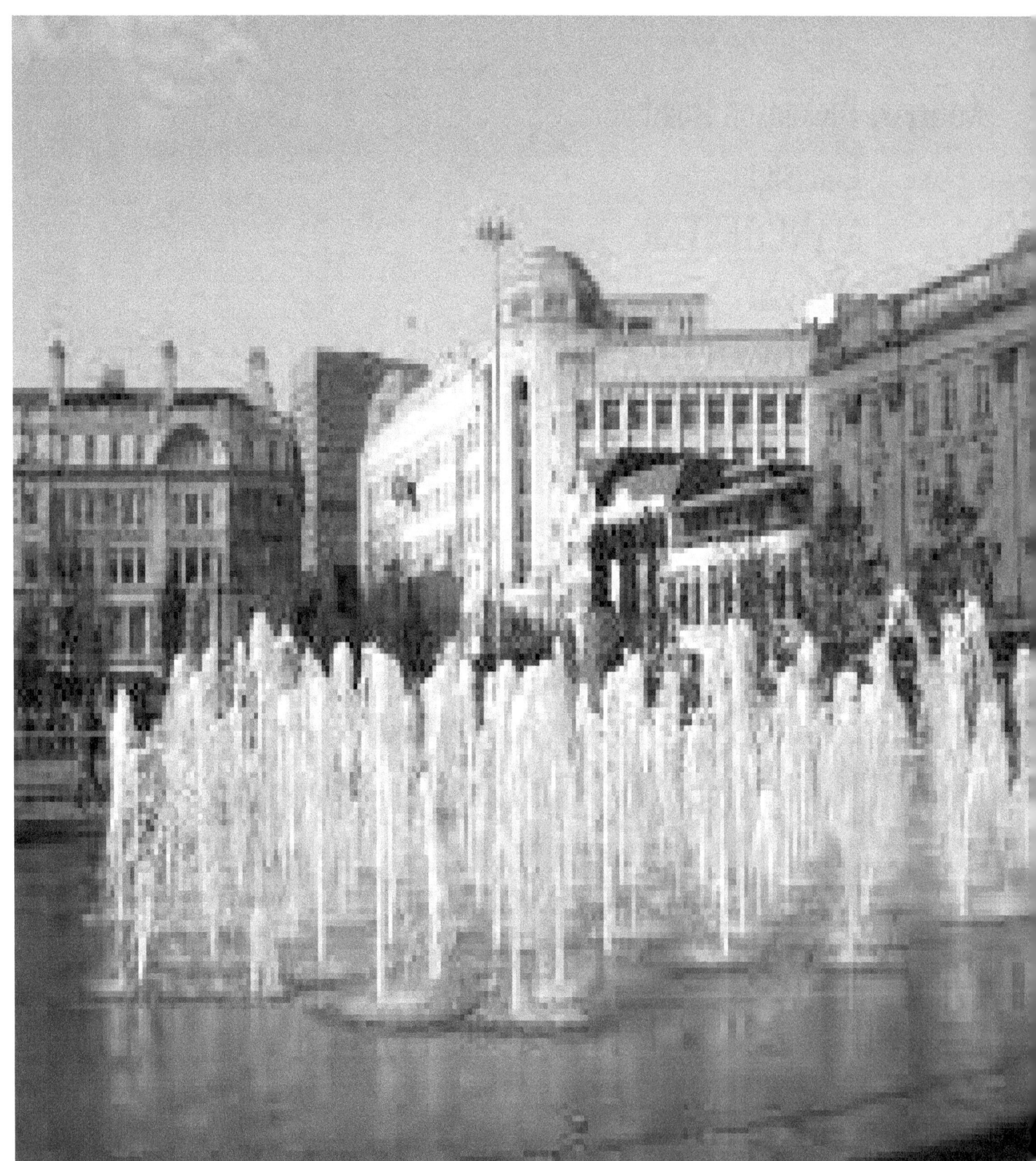

Booth drop in and activity centre

Address: Manchester Cathedral
Victoria Street
City Centre
MANCHESTER
M3 1SX

Contact: 0161 835 2499 Fax: 0161 839 6226
Email:amanda@croome.net
Web Address:www.boothcentre.org.uk

Services: Advocacy, Alcohol & Drugs, Befriending, Drop In / Day Centre, Employment / Training, Ethnic Minorities, Housing Service

Open: Mon-Fri 9:30am - 2:30pm but see website for programme of activities and drop-in times as these are regularly updated.

Restrictions: No alcohol and drugs on premises.

Carr Gomm Society

Address: 2nd Floor
        Paragon House
        48 Seymour Grove
        Old Trafford
        MANCHESTER
        M16 0LN

Contact: 0161 877 8847 Fax: 0161 877 8848
Email:info@carr-gomm.org.uk
Web Address:www.carr-gomm.org.uk

Services: Housing, care and support for single people with a range of needs. Employment / Training, Housing Service

Open: Mon-Fri 9am - 5pm

Restrictions: 16+ for some projects 18+ for some others

Creative Support

Address: 5th Floor
        Dale House
        35 Dale Street
        City Centre
        MANCHESTER
        M1 2HF

Contact: 0161 236 0829 Fax: 0161 237 5126
Email:enquiries@creativesupport.co.uk
Web Address:www.creativesupport.co.uk

Services: Supported housing, supported living and community support for people with mental health needs or learning disabilities

Open: Mon-Fri 9am - 8pm

Restrictions: Manchester residents. Self referral possible.

Lifeshare – Manchester

Address: 1st Floor
      27 Houldsworth Street
      City Centre
      MANCHESTER
      M1 1EH

Contact: 0161 235 0744 Fax: 0161 953 4001
email:office@lifeshare.co.uk web address:www.lifeshare.co.uk

Services: Advocacy, Alcohol & Drugs, Counselling, Housing Service, Self Help, Volunteering, Soup run in Piccadilly Gardens at 9pm every night

Open: Office hours 9am - 5pm

Manchester Next Step

Address: 49 Knutsford Road
Gorton
Manchester
M18 7NJ

Contact: 0161 223 7053 Fax: 0161 223 8992
email:nextstep@greatplaces.org.uk
web address:www.greatplaces.org.uk

Service: Housing Service, Mental Health Workers

OIpen: Mon - Sun 8.30 4.00

Restriction: Men aged 35 or over.

People First Housing Association

Address: 179 Royce Road
        Hulme
        Manchester
        M15 5TJ

Service: Housing related (floating) support for people of all ages in Manchester area and who have mental health problems.

Contact: 0161 226 1917 Fax: 0161 232 8422
email:admin@peoplefirsthousing.co.uk
web address:www.peoplefirsthousing.co.uk

Restriction: Referrals via telephone from organisations and self-referral.

Open: 9am - 5pm

Shelter - Greater Manchester Housing Aid Centre

Address: 5 Samuel Ogden Street
Manchester
M1 7AX

Contact: 0844 515 1640 email:manchester@shelter.org.uk
web address:www.shelter.org.uk

Service: Housing advice to tenants, homeowners and homeless people in Greater Manchester. Legal advice.

Open: Appointments available appointments must be made by phone.

Single Person's Resettlement Team (SPRT)

Contact: 0161 234 5340/ 07852 560573

Service: Support with accessing housing, and housing-related care-planning and support. People are allocated a support worker who will meet with them regularly

Open: 9-5 Monday to Friday

Restrictions: Clients can self-refer by telephone or be referred by agencies.

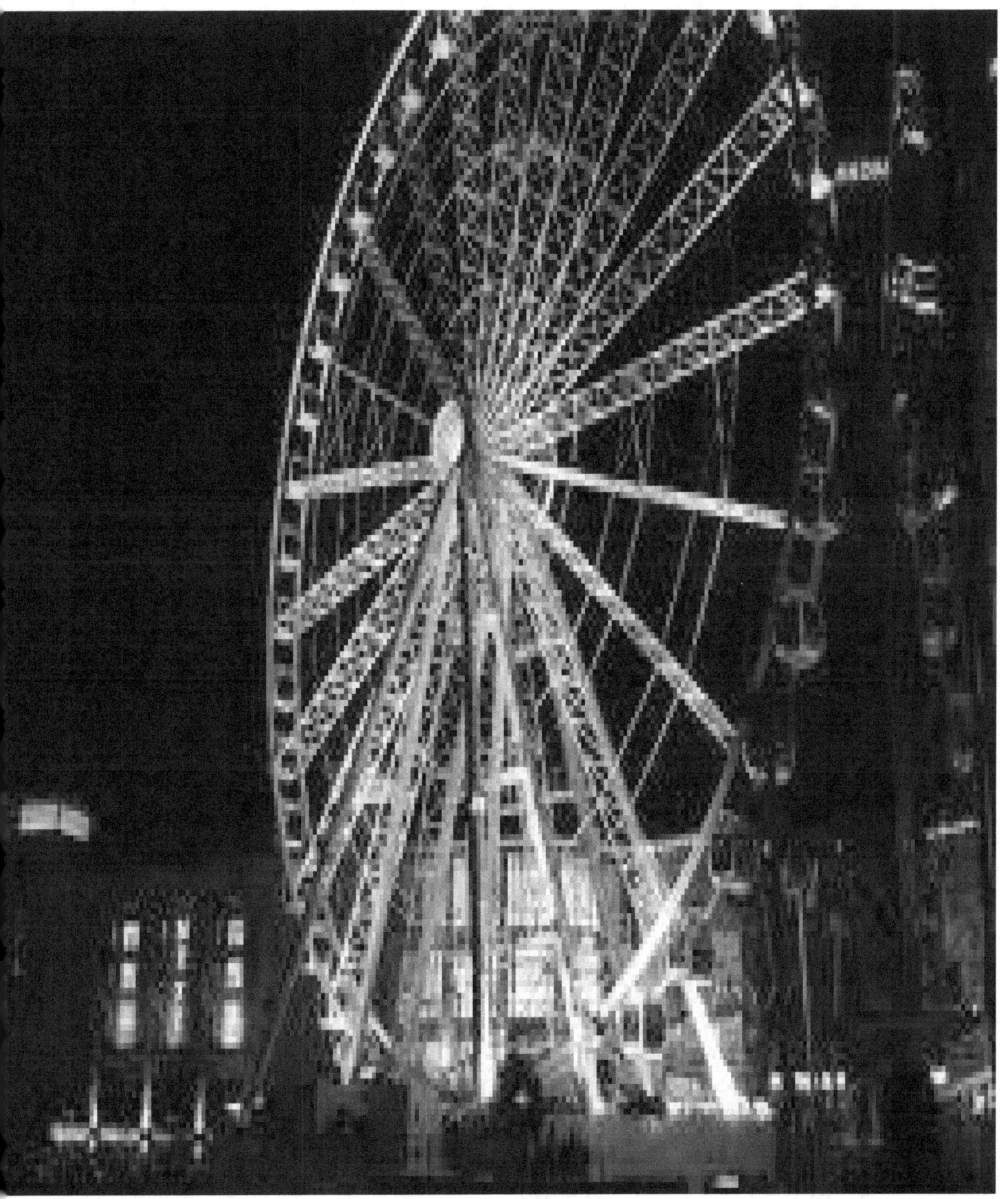

Contact Service for Social Care

Address: Manchester Contact Service
　　　Carisbrooke Resource Centre
　　　Wenlock Way
　　　West Gorton
　　　MANCHESTER
　　　M12 5LF

Contact: 0161 255 8250 (24hr emergencey number) Fax: 0161 255 8266 Minicom 0161 272 8787
Web Address:www.manchester.gov.uk/ssd/contact

Services: Alcohol & Drugs, Benefits / Welfare, Carers / Family, Depression, Disability, Ethnic Minorities, Housing Service, Learning Disability, Manic Depression / Bipolar, Older People, Schizophrenia, Self Harm, Young People

Open: 24hour/7day for emergencies
Restrictions: Manchester residents

Manchester Adult Placement Services

Address: 1st Floor
Crossacres Resource Centre
1 Peel Hall Road
Crossacres
Manchester
M22 5DG

Contact: 0161 437 3953 Fax: 0161 437 8831
email:donna.england@manchester.gov.uk
web address:www.manchester.gov.uk

Service: Adult Placement offers different types of care to vulnerable adults in the community, including those with mental health needs, physical disabilities and the elderly.

The care is provided by self employed approved providers either in their home or in the community.

Each provider is matched to the client based on personality or interests.

Open: 9am - 4:30pm

Restriction: Referrals by care manager only

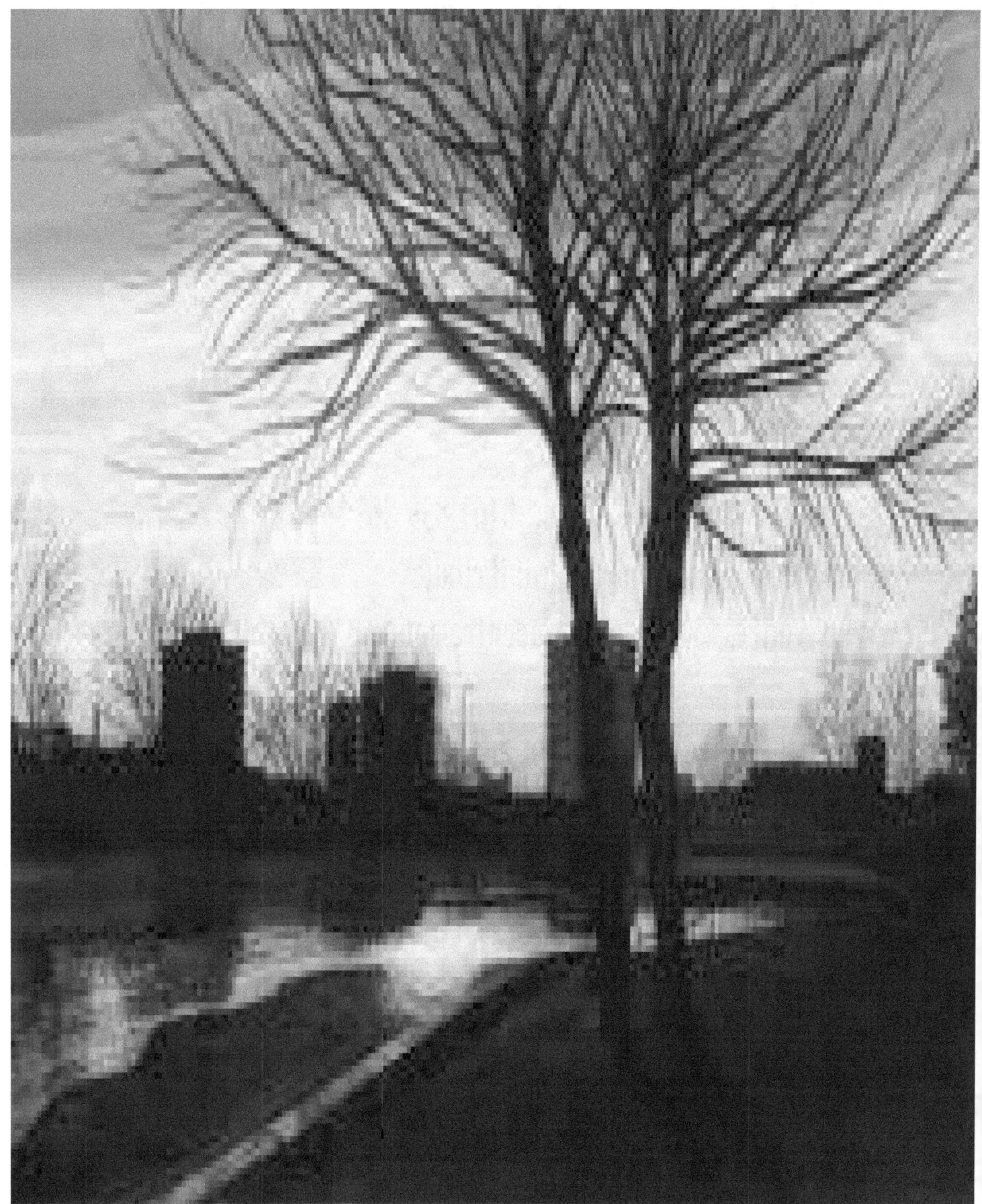

Carers Advice and info service

Address: Gaddum House
        6 Great Jackson Street
        City Centre
        MANCHESTER
        M15 4AX

Contact: 0161 834 6069 Fax: 0161 839 8574
Email:carersgaddum@hotmail.co.uk
Web Address:www.gaddumcentre.co.uk

Service: Advice, information and advocacy service for anyone who is concerned about care for their relatives

Open: Monday, Wednesday and Thursday office hours.

Restrictions: Manchester residents only

Development Project (National Autistic Society)

Address: Angelo House
Chapel Road
Northenden
Manchester
M22 4JN

Contact: Telephone: 0161 998 4667 Fax: 0161 945 2703
email:mari.saki@nas.org.uk web address:www.nas.org.uk

Services: The Family Services Development Project provides support to parents or other carers and individuals on the autistic spectrum, also works with staff from other agencies to improve the lives of people on the autistic spectrum

Open: Monday till Friday 9-5

Homestart Manchester

Address: River Park Trading Estate
River Park Road
Manchester
M40 2XP

Contact: 0161 230 6571/0800 0686368 Fax: 0161 223 8061
email:kathy.home-start@care4free.net
web address:www.homestartmc.org.uk

Service: Home-Start is a voluntary organisation in which volunteers offer regular support, friendship and practical help to young families under stress in their own homes, helping to prevent crisis and breakdown, and emphasing the pleasures of family life.

Any family with at least one child under five years of age may be referred to Home-Start for support if they are suffering stress or experiencing difficulties.

Referrals can be from health professionals or families themselves. 9am - 5pm for enquiries; some evening and weekend services provided for families with at least one child under 5

One parent families and Ginger Bread

Address: Room 2.2
Wind Rush Millemium Centre
70 Alexander Road
Moss Side
MANCHESTER
M16 7WD

Contact: 0161 636 7518 Fax: 0161 636 7564
email:info@oneparentfamilies.org.uk
web address:www.oneparentfamilies.org.uk

Service: Advice and counselling for single parents

Helpline 0800 018 5026 Helpline open Mon - Fri 9am-5pm and till 8pm on Weds

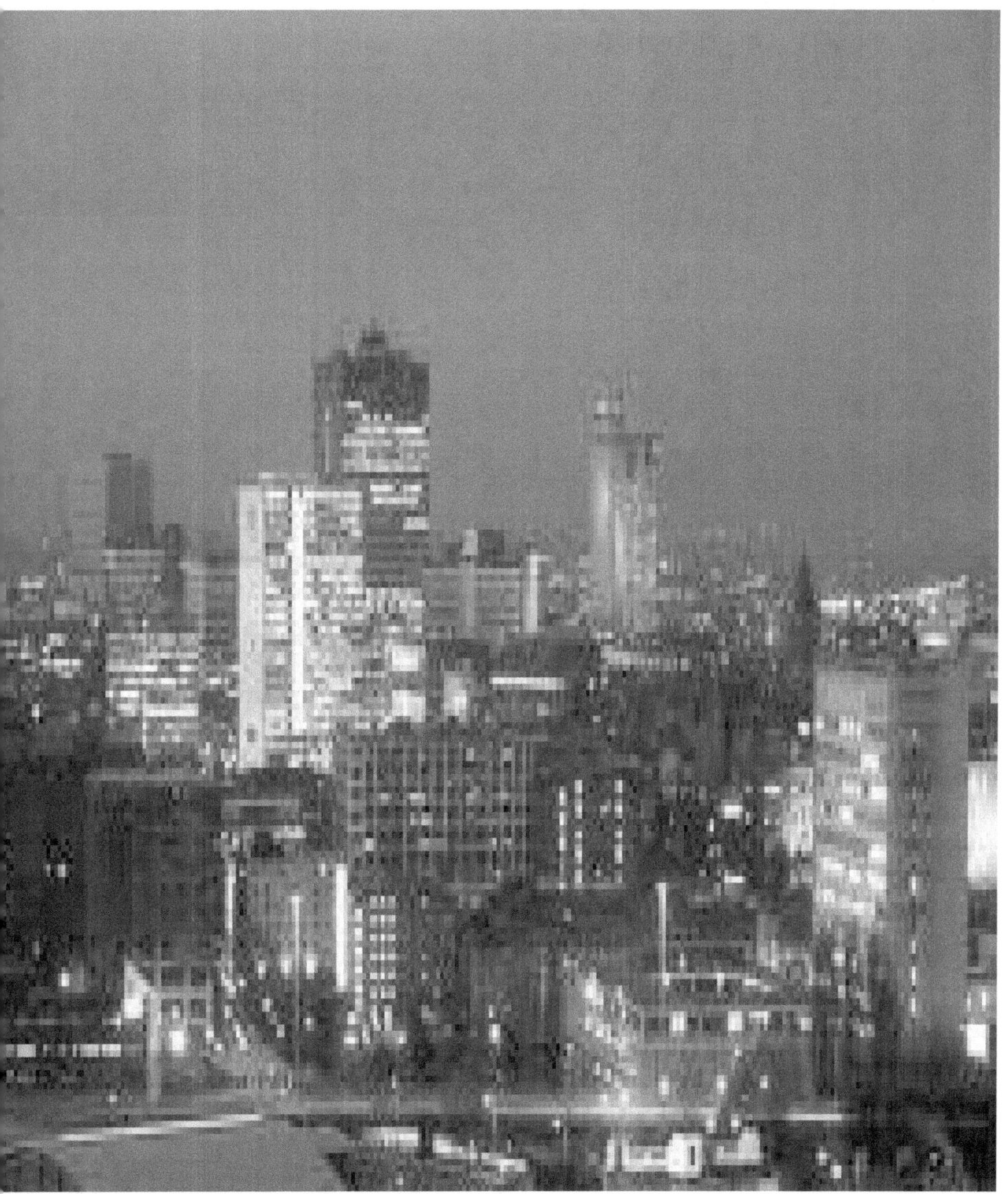

Cruse Bereavment Service

Address: Central Hall
         Oldham Street
         MANCHESTER
         M1 1JT

Contact: 0161 236 8103 Email:helpline@cruse.org.uk
Web Address:www.crusebereavementcare.org.uk

Bereavement counselling service Day by Day

 Helpline 0844 477 9400.

Young peron's freephone helpline 0808 808 1677

Open:.Mon-Fri 9.30- 5pm

North and South Manchester Counselling Service

Address: Woodville Resource Centre
Shirley Road
Cheetham Hill
MANCHESTER
M8 6NE

Contact: 07659 879593

Service: Confidential and non-judgemental counselling Self referrals only can be made. Leave details of your contact number and address on the answering machine and someone will contact you

Restriction: 18+

Relate - Greater Manchester South

Address: 346 Chester Rd
          Cornbrook
          MANCHESTER
          M16 9EZ

Contact: 0161 872 0303 Fax: 0161 877 7507
email:enquiries@relategms.co.uk
web address:www.relategms.co.uk

Service: Counselling, Gay Lesbian & Transgender, Older People, Young People, also families and relationship

Open: Mon-Fri 9am - 9:00pm, Sat 9am - 12 noon

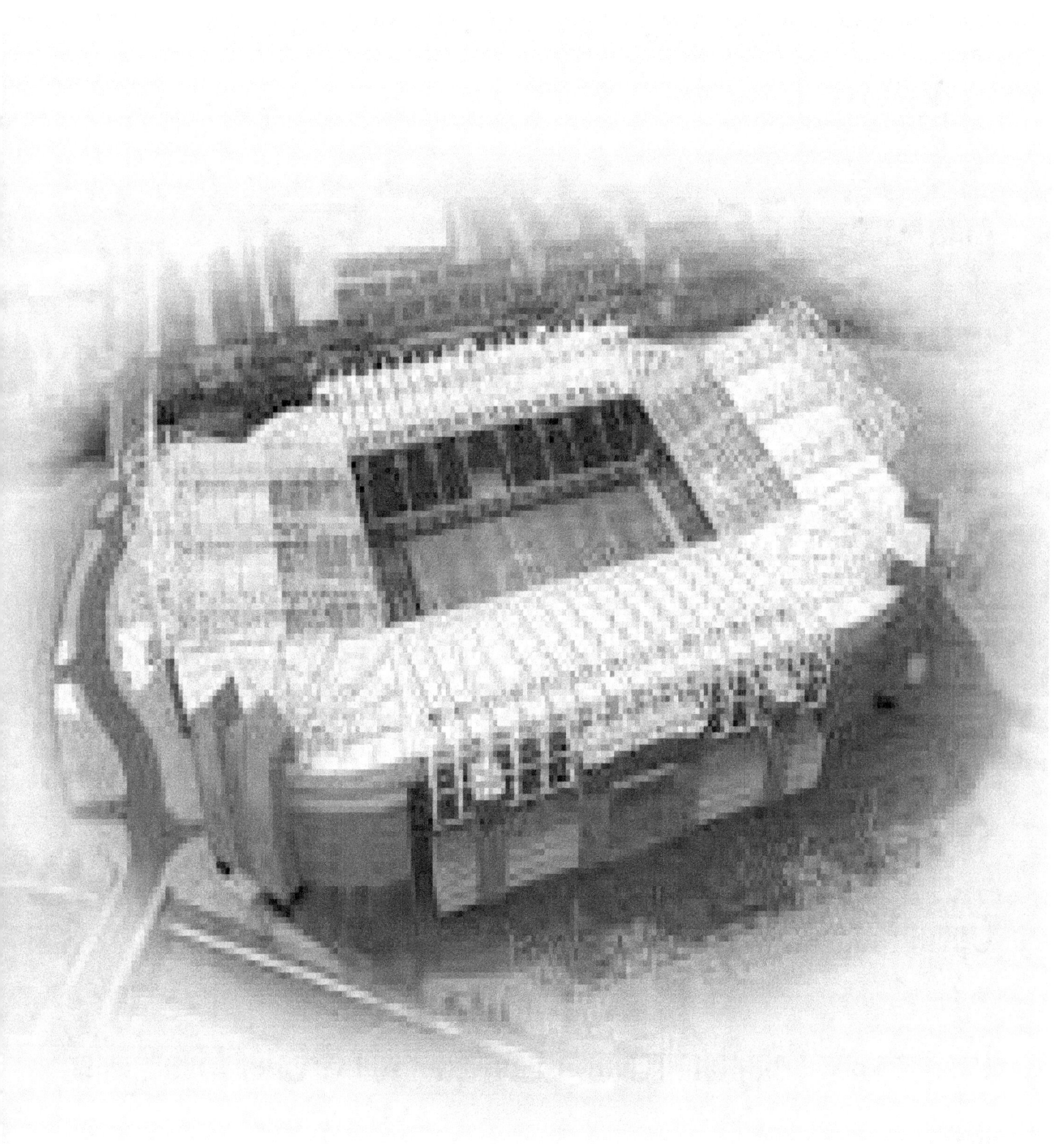

Greater Manchester Centre for Voluntary Organisations (GMCVO)

Address: St Thomas Centre

Ardwick Green North

MANCHESTER

M12 6FZ

Contact: 0161 277 1000 Fax: 0161 273 8296
email:gmcvo@gmcvo.org.uk web address: www.gmcvo.org.uk

Services: Provide training, consultancy, information, advice and practical support to voluntary organisations.

Open: Mon-Fri 10am - 4pm

Restrictions: Voluntary sector organisations in Greater Manchester area.

Head Forward Centre (Manchester)

Address: Withington Methodist Church
439 Wilmslow Road
Manchester
M20 4AN

Contact: 0161 434 2150
National helpline 0808 800 2244
email:headforward@tiscali.co.uk
web address:www.headforward.org

Services: Befriending, DisabilityDay centre

Open: Mon, Tues, Thurs & Fri 10 am to 3.30 pm.

Restriction: Attendance limited to 12 people. Daily attendance charge.